NUTRITION AND DIET RESEARCH PROGRESS

DIETS AND DISEASES

CAUSES AND PREVENTION

NUTRITION AND DIET RESEARCH PROGRESS

Additional books in this series can be found on Nova's website under the Series tab.

Additional e-books in this series can be found on Nova's website under the eBooks tab.

NUTRITION AND DIET RESEARCH PROGRESS

DIETS AND DISEASES

CAUSES AND PREVENTION

WENBIAO WU
EDITOR

New York

Additional color graphics may be available in the e-book version of this book.

Library of Congress Cataloging-in-Publication Data

ISBN: 978-1-63484-580-9
Library of Congress Control Number: 2015960801

Published by Nova Science Publishers, Inc. † New York

CONTENTS

PREFACE

The improvement of life expectance and quality is the primary target of modern society both in developed and developing countries. However, the global burden of diseases were estimated to be more than 2.74 billion DALYs with about 56.00 million global total deaths in 2012 by WHO. In 2030, the projected global burden of diseases and global total deaths are similar to or even higher than that in 2012. What are the causes of DALYs and deaths? What proportion do the causes contribute to global DALYS and deaths? Are global DALYS and deaths preventable? Are daily diets associated with global DALYs or deaths? What is the significance of diets contributing to global DALYs or deaths? Answers to these questions should be vital for the prevention and reduction of global DALYS and deaths.

More than 90% of causes contributing to the global total DALYs or deaths are modifiable or causable by daily diets. Therefore, understanding the association of diets with diseases is very necessary for us to reduce the global total DALYs or deaths in future.

Because of vast information about the diets and diseases in the literature, it is very difficult to collect them all in a limited space of a book within a limited time. This book opts to collect selected overview of association of diets with some important diseases.

Introduction – The significance of improper diets contributing to the global total DALYs or deaths is estimated by analyzing the existing data published by WHO. The conclusion is that diets should be critical factors that can modify or even cause the diseases, which significantly contribute to the global burden of diseases or deaths.

Chapter 1 - Twenty first century is described by a continuous progress in the field of food science: the discovery of nutrients, the guidelines for a healthy diet and the concept of a balanced diet gave to food development increasing dynamics. First came the power to eliminate malnutrition and later, an attempt to limit the excesses concerning the use of certain substances that are harmful to health. Nutritional sciences are ready to face new challenges, including those associated with the spread of the functional foods concept. A formal identification of functional food category is however quite complex, but in short functional foods may be considered technologically advanced and improved food products. These foods besides being in position to reduce the cost of healthcare from the aging population, could also give a commercial potential in the food industry.

Chapter 2 - Nutritional factors play critical roles in the development of cardiovascular diseases (CVD). There is a strong relationship between the reduction of CVD and the intake of plant-based foods and beverages. However, their effects on human health are still to be elucidated. Polyphenols from tea, coffee, and cacao have received much attention because they are known to have beneficial effects on CVD. The polyphenols in these beverages may reduce the risk of CVD through multiple mechanisms, including anti-oxidant and anti-inflammatory effects. This article reviews the evidence from experimental and clinical studies to show the potential effect of polyphenols from tea, coffee and cacao on the prevention of CVD.

Chapter 3 - The causes of kidney diseases are highlighted in this chapter. The risk factors, detection of the disease and diets suitable for managing kidney diseases are recommended. Foods that are low in potassium and phosphorus have been found suitable for managing early stages of kidney diseases. Food industries could develop novel food products from indigenous crops widely cultivated in each country where there is low in these minerals for people suffering from early stages of kidney diseases.

Chapter 4 - During menstrual cycle the body tends to crave certain foods, typically fatty, salty and/or sweet. For many, the association between diets and the reproductive system comes to stand still here. Yet, foods and diets are intricately linked to the reproductive system. What you eat, or fail to eat, can increase or decrease your chances of getting pregnant, worsen your PMS symptoms and possibly even disrupt your menstrual cycle. It is essential to get enough calcium. Women need at least 1,200 mg of calcium every day. Some good sources of calcium include low-fat milk, yogurt, broccoli and salmon. If milk is not in the diet, one can increase their calcium intake with soy or rice milk, tofu or kale. One must look for fermented soy products as certain soy products contain phytoestrogens, which can mimic the natural estrogen found in the body, leading to reproductive health difficulties. If there is too much or too little estrogen in your body, your fertility is significantly compromised. Men are different from women in all kinds of ways including their nutritional needs. Just as women need particular nutrients during pregnancy or for protection from breast cancer, men need nutrients that can help them maintain muscle mass, prevent prostate cancer, and more. Many foods that tend to be favorites among men are not the best choices for a good health. They can also enhance performance, from the board room to the bedroom.

Chapter 5 - Safe diet is very important for preventing human body from liver injury. The risk factors existing in human diets have been analyzed. Many risk factors of liver injury could be present in human diets.

It is concluded that our daily diets or foods contains several identified factors of damaging liver. These factors include over- or under-intake of some nutrients (including over-intake of energy, under-intake of protein/energy, over-intake of ethyl alcohol, over-intake of vitamin A, over-intake of niacin, over-intake of iron, over-intake of fluoride, and under- and over-intake of selenium), safrole, capsaicinoids, coumarin, gossypol, pyrrolizidine alkaloids, cycasin, heterocyclic amines, hydrazines, pyrones, pennyroyal oil, tannins, saponins, and contaminants.

Especially, over-intake of energy and under-intake of protein/energy are very significant because they are related to our staple foods or diets and therefore linked with daily diets or nutrition throughout life time. Heterocyclic amines are produced from meats during high temperature cooking. These risk factors are particular significant for people who are used to eat meats as staple foods and cook meats by grilling, frying or baking. The risk factors including over-intake of vitamin A, over-intake of niacin, over-intake of iron, over-intake of fluoride, and under- and over-intake of selenium could also be very significant because they are linked with daily diets or nutrition throughout life time. Tannins and saponins may have beneficial and adverse effect on health depending on their dosage. Others may be considered as toxins.

So many risk factors of liver injury could exist in foods. Their cooperative effects of the risk factors that are present in one's customary daily diet need to be studied well even though the concentration of each factor might be safe for consumption. Does any unknown risk factor of liver injury exist in foods?

Chapter 6 - The liver is the most complex and largest internal organ in the human body. It plays an important role in the maintenance of internal environment through its multiple and diverse functions. The liver is prone to various diseases as a result of its multidimensional function. The diseases are categorized into chronic and acute liver diseases. The burden of chronic liver disease is on the increase in both developed as well as developing countries. The main cause for this continuous rise of liver disease is non-alcoholic fatty liver disease (NAFLD). Hepatitis, another form of liver disease is also affecting millions of people worldwide. Though people survive with 70% liver damage, there is a substantial burden of morbidity from liver disease, a high cost to the National Health Scheme as well as a huge economic and human cost from liver related ill health.

Diets play significant roles in the management or development of liver diseases. Polyunsaturated fatty acids, proteins and minerals are important requirements in patients suffering from certain liver diseases. However, there are certain dietary related factors causing liver diseases such as obesity, protein-energy malnutrition, vitamin toxicity and aflatoxin exposure. Diets have also been found to confer hepatoprotective effecst on the liver from various studies especially diets high in antioxidant content, as several liver diseases are associated with oxidative stress. However despite these possibilities, antioxidants have produced mixed results in a number of clinical trials of efficacy. Dietary fatty acids have also been found to play important roles in the pathogenesis of liver diseases.

Consequently in this chapter, the causes, prevalence of different liver diseases are discussed, the role of consuming food grains with a high level of aflatoxin in the etiology of liver diseases and appropriate diets for prevention as part of management strategies of the different liver diseases are discussed.

Food industries are therefore urged to develop and produce appropriate nutritious food products for this category of the populace. In addition, food products meant for public consumption should be such that will not pose health risk such as for both acute and chronic liver diseases.

Chapter 7 - Nutrition related bone problems are very common in all nations across the globe. Over and under intake of certain nutrients is considered the major cause for these problems. Sometimes such problems may arise as a result of internal metabolites. This chapter will discuss the theories related to bone problems keeping in view the hypo and hyper conditions of nutrients in relation to bone related problems such as osteoporosis, osteomalacias, parathyroidism, Paget's disease, fibrous dysplasia and many more. Role of micro and macro minerals in relation to bone disease will also be the topic of discussion. Glimpses from previous research will be presented to gather the evidences that these problems can be well managed through the diet. Diet interaction with other factors such as genetic, medical, pharmacological and modern lifestyle will be viewed in relation to bone health. New techniques for evaluation of bone abnormalities will also be under discussion. Demographic data on bone disease will suggest who is more likely at risk. Finally, scientific strategies will be framed that will suggest some prophylactic measures intended to control the bone diseases through diets.

Chapter 8 - A detailed review of arthritis and their various forms, causes and symptoms are reported in this chapter. Diets that trigger arthritis, are enumerated and diets that could help to prevent, manage arthritis in addition to weight loss as well as physical exercises around the joints are proposed. Increasing daily consumption of foods rich in antioxidants and processed food products is suggested in preventing and managing arthritis.

Chapter 9 - A detailed review about the association of diet with overweight and obesity was extensively discussed in this chapter. The causes and symptoms of overweight and obesity, diet-related treatment of overweight and obesity, possible methods of reducing obesity and overweight are being proposed at individual levels and via research and development as well as through the food industries in form of production of healthy food products such as high fibre meals, snacks, drinks etc. Nutritional campaign or education against overweight and obesity needs to be conducted particularly in most developing countries in Africa.

Chapter 10 - When people eat healthily, they feel healthy, work better, they have an increased performance at work and they become happy as they feel socially well. Human body requires foods consumed externally in order to function properly. If we take more than enough calories or the body doesn't burn enough calorie, body starts to store the extra energy. Today, fast-food products which are consumed largely by children or young people can cause lack of nutrition or malnutrition and therefore, they increase the risk of obesity. Obesity defined as the excessive fat tissue in the body affects over 300 million people according to the data of World Health Organization (WHO). Obesity spreads like an epidemic and it also becomes an economical burden by increasing health expenses of the countries. Nearly a billion people are obese.

Obesity is a serious health problem which causes various disorders through effecting mainly cardiovascular and endocrine system and it can even cause death. There are many factors effecting development of obesity; demographic factors, genetic susceptibility, environmental factors, behavioral factors, diet, eating habits and psychological factors are the most significant reasons of obesity. In the present study, these causes of obesity will be handled and behavioral factors, diet and eating habits will be examined in detail. In obesity disorder developed by wrong or unbalanced eating habits fat cell formation is very fast especially in the first few years of the life. The number of fat cells increases when fat storage becomes faster in the body. The number of fat cells for the obese children is three times more than normal weight children. Obese children diet indicates that they take extra energy from the fat. Eating style in babyhood determines the eating habits of a child later in life. Eating fast and chewing less are among the factors easing development of obesity.

Efforts to avoid obesity are the essence of fighting against this disease. In this respect, what is important is not to cure obesity well but to avoid it. Thus, starting from the fetal period, proper eating habits should be developed.

INTRODUCTION

Wenbiao Wu[1,*] and Yiqun Wang[2]

[1]College of Food Science, Southwest University, Chongqing, PRC

[2]Department of Medicine, Imperial College, London, UK

The improvement of life expectance and quality is the primary target of modern society both in developed and developing countries. To achieve this target, it is necessary to find or understand the critical and determinant factors of the life expectance and quality. What is the indicative index of the life expectance and quality? The rate of global total disability-adjusted life years (DALYs; a measurement of global burden of diseases) and deaths in the world is primarily employed in indicating global life expectance and quality.

World Health Organization frequently produces and updates the data and statistics of global DALYs and deaths. In 2004, the global DALYs and deaths were reported to be just over 1.53 billion and 58.77 million, respectively (1). The global DALYs were reported to be more than 2.74 billion while the global total deaths were about 56.00 million in 2012 (2). The global total deaths were projected to be just over 57.32 million in 2015 while they may be up to more than 70.10 million in 2030 (3). Arising from these data and statistics published, it stands reasons to ask several important and useful questions.

What are the causes of DALYs and deaths? What proportion do the causes contribute to global DALYS and deaths? Are global DALYS and deaths preventable? Are daily diets associated with global DALYs or deaths? What is the significance of diets contributing to global DALYs or deaths? Answers to these questions should be vital for the prevention and reduction of global DALYS and deaths. The aim of this chapter is therefore to answer these questions.

CAUSES OF GLOBAL DALYS AND DEATHS

In general, the potential causes of global DALYs and deaths may include viral or bacterial infection, physical damage, genetic inheritance or mutation, intake of toxic

*Corresponding Author Address: College of Food Science, Southwest University, 216 Tian Sheng Qiao, Beibei, Chongqing, PRC Email: wbwu62@yahoo.com.

compounds, over- or under-intake of essential nutrients or an unbalanced diet (4,5). The exact causes of were global DALYs and deaths were counted and included in WHO's data and statistical bank. The major parts of causes of DALYs result in deaths. They were also projected for the future years.

For example, according to WHO's data and statistical bank in 2012, the causes of global DALYs can be classified as the following:

1. communicable, maternal, perinatal and nutritional diseases;
2. noncommunicable diseases;
3. injuries.

The first group of causes can be further subdivided into:

1. infectious and parasitic diseases which include tuberculosis, STDS excluding HIV (including syphilis, chlamydia, gonorrhoea, trichomoniasis, and other STDs), HIV/AIDS, diarrhoeal diseases, childhood-cluster diseases (including whooping cough, diphtheria, measles, and tetanus), meningitis, encephalitis, acute hepatitis B, acute hepatitis C, parasitic and vector diseases (including malaria, trypanosomiasis, chagas disease, schistosomiasis, leishmaniasis, lymphatic filariasis, onchocerciasis, leprosy, dengue, trachoma, and rabies), intestine nematode infections (ascariasis, trichuriasis, and hookworm diseases), and other infectious diseases;
2. respiratory infections which include lower respiratory infections, upper respiratory infections, and otitis media;
3. maternal conditions;
4. neonatal conditions which include preterm birth complications, birth asphyxia and birth trauma, neonatal sepsis and infections, and other neonatal conditions;
5. nutritional deficiencies which include protein-energy malnutrition, iodine deficiency, vitamin A deficiency, iron-deficiency anaemia, and other nutritional deficiencies.

The second group of causes can be further subdivided into:

1. malignant neoplasms which include mouth and oropharynx cancers, oesophagus cancers, stomach cancer, colon and rectum cancers, liver cancer, pancreas cancer, trachea, bronchus and lung cancers, melanoma and other skin cancers, breast cancer, cervix uteri cancer, corpus uteri cancer, ovary cancer, prostate cancer, bladder cancer, lymphomas and multiple myeloma, leukaemia, and other malignant neoplasms;
2. other neoplasms;
3. diabetes mellitus;
4. endocrine, blood and immune disorders;
5. mental and behavioral disorders which include unipolar depressive disorders, bipolar disorders, schizophrenia, alcohol use disorders, drug use disorders, anxiety disorders, eating disorders, pervasive developmental disorders, childhood behavioral disorders, idiopathic intellectual disability, and other mental and behavioral disorders;

6. neurological conditions which include Alzheimer's disease and other dementias, Parkinson's disease, epilepsy, multiple sclerosis, migraine, non-migraine headache, and other neurological conditions;
7. sense organ diseases which include glaucoma, cataracts, refractive errors, macular degeneration, other vision loss, other hearing loss, and other sense organ diseases;
8. cardiovascular diseases which include rheumatic heart disease, hypertensive heart disease, ischaemic heart disease, stroke, cardiomyopathy, myocarditis, endocarditis, and other circulating diseases;
9. respiratory diseases which include chronic obstructive pulmonary disease, asthma, and other respiratory diseases;
10. digestive diseases which include peptic ulcer disease, cirrhosis of the liver, appendicitis, and other digestive diseases;
11. genitourinary diseases which include kidney diseases, hyperplasia of prostate, urolithiasis, other genitourinary diseases, infertility, and gynecological diseases;
12. skin diseases;
13. musculoskeletal diseases which include rheumatoid arthritis, osteoarthritis, gout, beck and neck pain, and other musculoskeletal disorders;
14. congenital anomalies which include neural tube defects, cleft lip and cleft palate, Down's syndrome, congenital heart anomalies, other chromosomal anomalies, and other congenital anomalies;
15. oral conditions which include dental caries, periodontal disease, and edentulism.

The third group can be further subdivided into:

1. unintentional injuries which include road injury, poisonings, falls, fire, heat and hot substances, drowning, exposure to forces of nature, and other unintentional injuries;
2. intentional injuries which include self harm, interpersonal violence, and collective violence and legal intervention.

According to WHO's projections, the potential causes of global deaths in 2030 can be classified as the following:

1. communicable, maternal, perinatal and nutritional diseases;
2. noncommunicable diseases;
3. injuries.

The first group of causes can be further subdivided into:

1. infectious and parasitic diseases which include tuberculosis, STDS excluding HIV (including syphilis, chlamydia, gonorrhoea, and other STDs), HIV/AIDS, diarrhoeal diseases, childhood-cluster diseases (including whooping cough, diphtheria, measles, and tetanus), meningitis, encephalitis, acute hepatitis B, acute hepatitis C, parasitic and vector diseases (including malaria, trypanosomiasis, chagas disease, schistosomiasis, leishmaniasis, lymphatic filariasis, leprosy, dengue, trachoma, and rabies), intestine nematode infections (ascariasis, and hookworm diseases), and other infectious diseases;

2. respiratory infections which include lower respiratory infections, upper respiratory infections, and otitis media;
3. maternal conditions;
4. neonatal conditions which include preterm birth complications, birth asphyxia and birth trauma, neonatal sepsis and infections, and other neonatal conditions;
5. nutritional deficiencies which include protein-energy malnutrition, iodine deficiency, vitamin A deficiency, iron-deficiency anaemia, and other nutritional deficiencies.

The second group of causes can be further subdivided into:

1. malignant neoplasms which include mouth and oropharynx cancers, oesophagus cancers, stomach cancer, colon and rectum cancers, liver cancer, pancreas cancer, trachea, bronchus and lung cancers, melanoma and other skin cancers, breast cancer, cervix uteri cancer, corpus uteri cancer, ovary cancer, prostate cancer, bladder cancer, lymphomas and multiple myeloma, leukaemia and other malignant neoplasms;
2. other neoplasms;
3. diabetes mellitus;
4. endocrine, blood and immune disorders;
5. mental and behavioral disorders which include unipolar depressive disorders, bipolar disorder, schizophrenia, alcohol use disorders, drug use disorders, anxiety disorders, pervasive developmental disorders, eating disorders, idiopathic intellectual disability, and other mental and behavioral disorders;
6. neurological conditions which include Alzheimer's disease and other dementias, Parkinson's disease, epilepsy, multiple sclerosis, migraine, non-migraine headache and other neurological conditions;
7. sense organ diseases which include glaucoma, cataracts, other hearing loss, and other sense organ diseases;
8. cardiovascular diseases which include rheumatic heart disease, hypertensive heart disease, ischaemic heart disease, stroke, cardiomyopathy, myocarditis, endocarditis, and other circulating diseases;
9. respiratory diseases which include chronic obstructive pulmonary disease, asthma, and other respiratory diseases;
10. digestive diseases which include peptic ulcer disease, cirrhosis of the liver, appendicitis, and other digestive diseases;
11. genitourinary diseases which include kidney diseases, hyperplasia of prostate, urolithiasis, other genitourinary diseases, and gynecological diseases;
12. skin diseases;
13. musculoskeletal diseases which include rheumatoid arthritis, osteoarthritis, gout, beck and neck pain, and other musculoskeletal disorders;
14. congenital anomalies which include neural tube defects, cleft lip and cleft palate, Down's syndrome, congenital heart anomalies, other chromosomal anomalies, and other congenital anomalies;
15. oral conditions which include dental caries, periodontal disease, and edentulism.

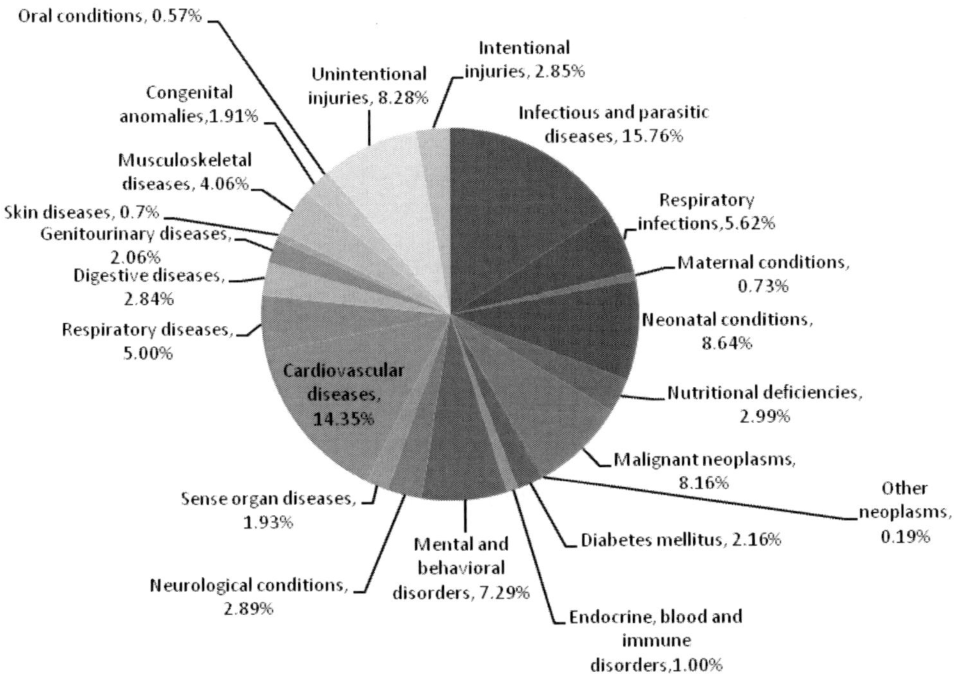

Figure 1. Percentage of causes contributing to that (100%) of global total DALYs in 2012.

The third group can be further subdivided into:

1. unintentional injuries which include road injury, poisonings, falls, fire, heat and hot substances, drowning, and other unintentional injuries;
2. intentional injuries which include self harm, interpersonal violence, and collective violence and legal intervention.

Percentage of Causes Contributing to Global DALYs and Deaths

As mentioned just in the above section, there are so many causes contributing to the global DALYs and deaths. However, the majority of DALYs and deaths are mainly contributed by only limited proportion of all causes.

Percentage of Causes Contributing to Global DALYs

Figure 1 shows the percentage of causes contributing the global total DALYs in 2012. The percentage of infections and parasitic diseases subgroup contributing to the global total DALYs is the largest among that of all causes. Ranking all varieties of infectious and parasitic diseases subgroup in the order of contribution to the global total DALYs, it would be as the following: diarrhoeal diseases > HIV/AIDS > parasitic and vector diseases (including malaria, trypanosomiasis, chagas disease, schistosomiasis, leishmaniasis, lymphatic filariasis, onchocerciasis, leprosy, dengue, trachoma, and rabies) > tuberculosis > other infectious diseases > meningitis > childhood-cluster diseases (including whooping cough, diphtheria, measles, and tetanus) > STDS excluding HIV (including syphilis, chlamydia, gonorrhoea, and other STDs) > acute hepatitis B > encephalitis > intestine nematode infections (ascariasis, trichuriasis, and hookworm diseases) > acute hepatitis C. The percentage of cardiovascular diseases subgroup contributing to the global total DALYs is the second largest among that of all causes. Ranking all varieties of cardiovascular diseases subgroup in the order of contribution to the global total DALYs, it would be as the following: ischaemic heart disease > stroke > other circulating diseases > hypertensive heart disease > cardiomyopathy, myocarditis, and endocarditis > rheumatic heart disease. The percentage of neonatal conditions subgroup contributing to the global total DALYs is the third largest among that of all causes. The percentage of unintentional injuries subgroup contributing to the global total DALYs is the fourth largest among that of all causes. The percentage of malignant neoplasms subgroup contributing to the global total DALYs is the fifth largest among that of all causes. Ranking all varieties of malignant neoplasms subgroup in the order of contribution to the global total DALYs, it would be as the following: trachea, bronchus and lung cancers > other malignant neoplasms > liver cancer > stomach cancer > breast cancer > colon and rectum cancers > leukaemia > oesophagus cancers > mouth and oropharynx cancers > cervix uteri cancer = lymphomas and multiple myeloma > pancreas cancer > prostate cancer > ovary cancer > bladder cancer > melanoma and other skin cancers > corpus uteri cancer. The percentage of mental and behavioral disorders subgroup contributing to the global total DALYs is the sixth largest among that of all causes. Ranking all varieties of mental and behavioral disorders subgroup in the order of contribution to the global total DALYs, it would be as the following: unipolar depressive disorders > alcohol use disorders > anxiety disorders > drug use disorders > schizophrenia > bipolar disorder > pervasive developmental disorders > idiopathic intellectual disability > eating disorders > other mental and behavioral disorders. The percentage of respiratory infections subgroup contributing to the global total DALYs is the seventh largest among that of all causes. Ranking all varieties of respiratory infections subgroup in the order of contribution to the global total DALYs, it would be as the following: lower respiratory infections > otitis media > upper respiratory infections. The percentage of respiratory diseases subgroup contributing to the global total DALYs is the eighth largest among that of all causes. Ranking all varieties of respiratory diseases subgroup in the order of contribution to the global total DALYs, it would be as the following: chronic obstructive pulmonary disease > asthma > other respiratory diseases. The percentage of musculoskeletal diseases subgroup contributing to the global total DALYs is the ninth largest among that of all causes. Ranking all varieties of musculoskeletal diseases subgroup in the order of contribution to the global total DALYs, it would be as the following: beck and neck pain > other musculoskeletal disorders> osteoarthritis> rheumatoid arthritis > gout. The percentage of nutritional deficiencies subgroup contributing to the global total DALYs is the tenth largest among that of all causes. Ranking all varieties of nutritional deficiencies subgroup in the order of contribution to the global total DALYs, it would be as the following: iron-deficiency anaemia > protein-energy malnutrition > iodine deficiency > vitamin A deficiency > other nutritional deficiencies. Ranking all other diseases subgroups in the order of contribution to the global total DALYs, it would be as the following: neurological conditions > intentional injuries > digestive diseases > diabetes mellitus > genitourinary diseases > sense organ diseases > congenital anomalies > endocrine, blood and immune disorders > maternal conditions > skin diseases > oral conditions > other neoplasms.

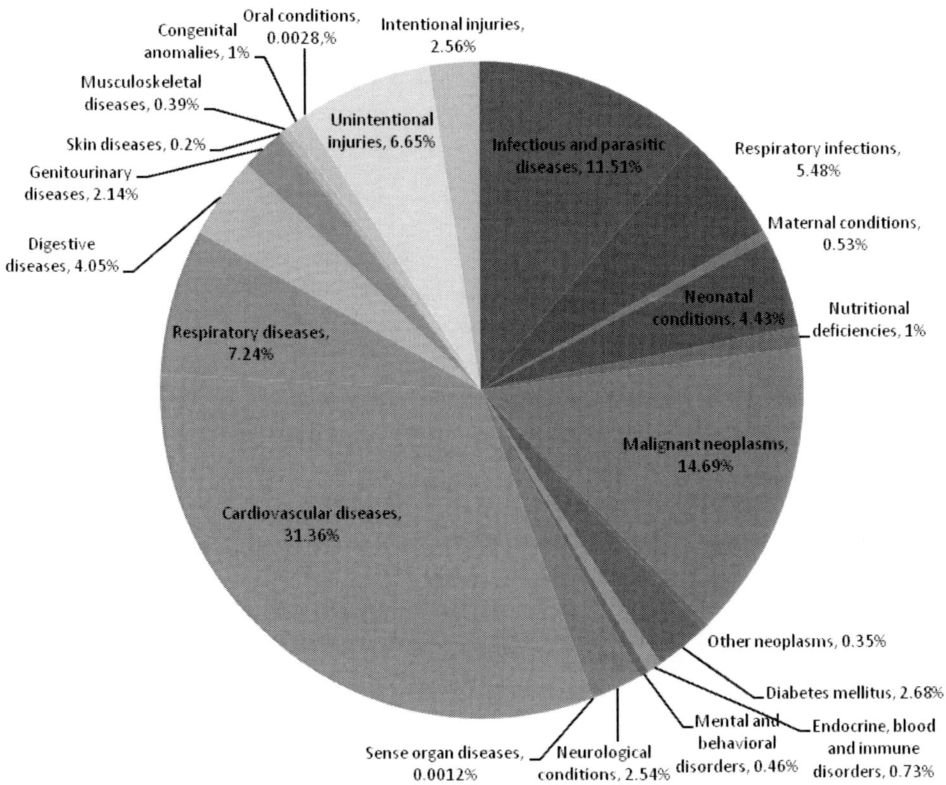

Figure 2. Projected percentage of causes contributing to that (100%) of global total deaths in 2012. The percentage of each cause was calculated by using the data published by WHO (6).

Percentage of Causes Contributing to Global Deaths

Figure 2 shows the percentage of causes (subgroups) contributing the global total deaths in 2012. Ranking all diseases (subgroups) in the order of contribution to the global total deaths, it would be as the following: cardiovascular diseases > malignant neoplasms > infectious and parasitic diseases > respiratory diseases > unintentional injuries > respiratory infections > neonatal conditions > digestive diseases > diabetes mellitus > intentional injuries > neurological conditions > genitourinary diseases > nutritional deficiencies = congenital anomalies > endocrine, blood and immune disorders > maternal conditions > mental and behavioral disorders > musculoskeletal diseases > other neoplasms > skin diseases > oral conditions > sense organ diseases.

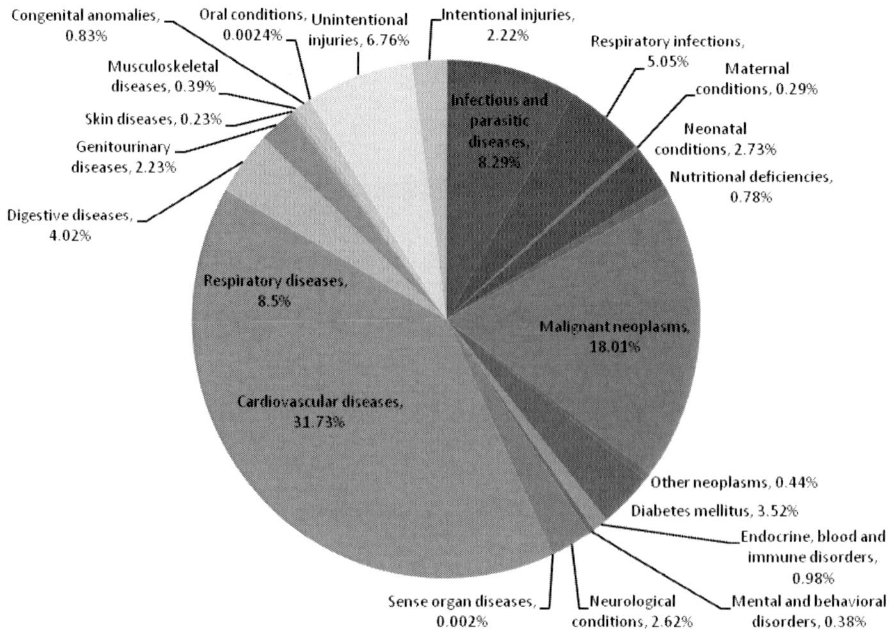

Figure 3. Projected percentage of causes contributing to that (100%) of global total deaths in 2030. The percentage of each cause was calculated by using the data published by WHO (3).

Figure 3 shows the projected percentage of causes (subgroups) contributing the global total deaths in 2030. The percentage of cardiovascular diseases subgroup contributing to the global total deaths is the largest among that of all causes. Ranking all varieties of cardiovascular diseases subgroup in the order of contribution to the global total deaths, it would be as the following: ischaemic heart disease > stroke > other circulating diseases > hypertensive heart disease > cardiomyopathy, myocarditis, and endocarditis > rheumatic heart disease. The percentage of malignant neoplasms subgroup contributing to the global total deaths is the second largest among that of all causes. Ranking all varieties of malignant neoplasms subgroup in the order of contribution to the global total deaths, it would be as the following: trachea, bronchus and lung cancers > other malignant neoplasms > liver cancer > stomach cancer > colon and rectum cancers > breast cancer > oesophagus cancers > prostate cancer > lymphomas and multiple myeloma > mouth and oropharynx cancers > pancreas cancer > cervix uteri cancer > leukaemia > bladder cancer > ovary cancer > melanoma and other skin cancers > corpus uteri cancer. The percentage of respiratory diseases subgroup contributing to the global total deaths is the third largest among that of all causes. Ranking all varieties of respiratory diseases subgroup in the order of contribution to the global total deaths, it would be as the following: chronic obstructive pulmonary disease > other respiratory diseases > asthma. The percentage of infectious and parasitic diseases subgroup contributing to the global total deaths is the fourth largest among that of all causes. Ranking all varieties of infectious and parasitic diseases subgroup in the order of contribution to the global total deaths, it would be as the following: HIV/AIDS > diarrhoeal diseases > tuberculosis > parasitic and vector diseases (including malaria, trypanosomiasis, chagas disease, schistosomiasis, leishmaniasis, lymphatic filariasis, leprosy, dengue, trachoma, and rabies) > other infectious diseases > acute hepatitis C > meningitis > acute hepatitis B >

childhood-cluster diseases (including whooping cough, diphtheria, measles, and tetanus) > encephalitis > STDS excluding HIV (including syphilis, chlamydia, gonorrhoea, and other STDs) > intestine nematode infections (ascariasis, and hookworm diseases). The percentage of unintentional injuries subgroup contributing to the global total deaths is the sixth largest among that of all causes. Ranking all varieties of unintentional injuries subgroup in the order of contribution to the global total deaths, it would be as the following: road injury > other unintentional injuries > falls > drowning > fire, heat and hot substances > poisonings. The percentage of digestive diseases subgroup contributing to the global total deaths is the seventh largest among that of all causes. Ranking all varieties of digestive diseases subgroup in the order of contribution to the global total deaths, it would be as the following: other digestive diseases > cirrhosis of the liver > peptic ulcer disease > appendicitis. The percentage of diabetes mellitus subgroup contributing to the global total deaths is the eighth largest among that of all causes. The percentage of neonatal conditions subgroup contributing to the global total deaths is the ninth largest among that of all causes. Ranking all varieties of neonatal conditions subgroup in the order of contribution to the global total deaths, it would be as the following: preterm birth complications > birth asphyxia and birth trauma > neonatal sepsis and infections > other neonatal conditions. The percentage of neurological conditions subgroup contributing to the global total deaths is the tenth largest among that of all causes. Ranking all varieties of neurological conditions subgroup in the order of contribution to the global total deaths, it would be as the following: Alzheimer's disease and other dementias > other neurological conditions > epilepsy > Parkinson's disease > multiple sclerosis > migraine. Ranking all other diseases subgroups in the order of contribution to the global total deaths, it would be as the following: genitourinary diseases > intentional injuries > endocrine, blood and immune disorders > congenital anomalies > nutritional deficiencies > other neoplasms > musculoskeletal diseases > mental and behavioral disorders > maternal conditions > skin diseases > oral conditions > sense organ diseases.

Table 1 shows the comparison between the percentage of causes contributing to the global total deaths in 2012 and that projected in 2030. From 2012 to 2030, the global total deaths has been projected to significantly increase. Also, from 2012 to 2030, the percentage of cardiovascular diseases, malignant neoplasms, respiratory diseases, unintentional injuries, diabetes mellitus, neurological conditions, genitourinary diseases, endocrine, blood and immune disorders, other neoplasms and sense organ diseases contributing to the global total deaths has been estimated to increase while that of other diseases has been predicted to decrease.

Significance of Diets Contributing to Global DALYs and Deaths

What significance are daily diets associated with global DALYs or deaths? Common foods in daily diets can supply nutrients that are essential for the growth and maintenance of human body. Therefore, they should be significantly associated with diseases that are caused by nutritional deficiencies. Also, since foods are not just pure essential nutrients, they usually contain many components which are not essential nutrients. Some of these components could be functional whereas some others could be toxic. They could be vital for reducing or increasing diseases.

Table 1. Comparison between the percentage of causes contributing to the global total deaths in 2012 and that projected in 2030*

Type of cause	2012	2030
All causes deaths (person)	55,858,719	70,103,996
Cardiovascular diseases	31.36%	31.73%
Malignant neoplasms	14.69%	18.01%
Infectious and parasitic diseases	11.51	8.29%
Respiratory diseases	7.24%	8.50%
Unintentional injuries	6.65%	6.76%
Neonatal conditions	4.43%	2.73%
Digestive diseases	4.05%	4.02%
Diabetes mellitus	2.68%	3.52%
Intentional injuries	2.56%	2.22%
Neurological conditions	2.54%	2.62%
Genitourinary diseases	2.14%	2.23%
Nutritional deficiencies	1.00%	0.78%
Congenital anomalies	1.00%	0.83%
Endocrine, blood, immune disorders	0.73%	0.98%
Maternal conditions	0.53%	0.29%
Mental and behavioral disorders	0.46%	0.38%
Musculoskeletal diseases	0.39%	0.39%
Other neoplasms	0.35%	0.44%
Skin diseases	0.20%	0.23%
Oral conditions	0.028‰	0.024‰
Sense organ diseases	0.012‰	0.020‰

*Data sources: WHO (2, 3).

Significance of Nutritional Deficiencies

Nutritional deficiencies subgroup contributed to 2.99% of the global total DALYs in 2012, which was the tenth largest cause among all causes (2). The varieties of nutritional deficiencies subgroup included iron-deficiency anaemia, protein-energy malnutrition, iodine deficiency, vitamin A deficiency, and other nutritional deficiencies which contributed to 1.74%, 1.04%, 0.15%, 0.56‰, and 0.097‰ of global total DALYs, respectively.

Nutritional deficiencies subgroup contributed to 1.00% of global total deaths in 2012, which was the fifth largest cause among all causes (3). The varieties of the nutritional deficiency subgroup include protein-energy malnutrition, iron-deficiency anaemia, other nutritional deficiencies, iodine deficiency, and vitamin A deficiency which contributed to 0.82%, 0.16%, 0.16‰, 0.058‰, and 2.16×10^{-3}‰ of global total deaths, respectively. Although the projected percentage of the nutritional deficiencies subgroup contributing to the global total deaths in 2030 is slightly lower, comparing with that in 2012, it is still significant (3).

Significance of Diets Contributing to Other Varieties of DALYs and Deaths

Association of Diets with Injuries

Figure 1 indicates that injuries (unintentional + intentional) contributed to 11.14% of the global total DALYs in 2012. Poisoning (one variety of injuries) contributed to 0.39% of the global total DALYs. The poisoning is causable by toxins that are present in improper diets. Also, intentional injuries might be modifiable with improper diets for example the presence of excessive amount of depressing or agitating compounds. Therefore, only unintentional injuries except for poisoning cannot be caused by improper diets. This means that only 7.85% of the global total DALYs in 2012 caused by injuries cannot be caused by improper diets.

Figure 2 shows that injuries (unintentional + intentional) contributed to 9.21% of the global total deaths in 2012. Poisoning (one variety of injuries) contributed to 0.35% of the global total deaths. Similar to the reasons just mentioned in the above paragraph, the poisoning can be caused by toxins that are present in improper diets. Only unintentional injuries (only contributed to 6.30% of the global total deaths in 2012) except for poisoning cannot be caused by improper diets.

Figure 3 indicates that the projected injuries (unintentional + intentional) will contribute to 8.98% of the global total deaths in 2030. Poisoning (one variety of injuries) contributed to 0.28% of the global total deaths. Similar to the reasons just mentioned in the above two paragraphs, Only unintentional injuries (only projected contribution to 6.48% of the global total deaths in 2030) except for poisoning cannot be caused by improper diets.

It is therefore estimated that injuries contributed to 3.29% the global total DALYs in 2012 can be caused by improper diets. It is also estimated that injuries contributed to 2.91% the global total deaths in 2012 cannot be caused by improper diets. Furthermore, injuries projected a contribution of 2.50% to the global total deaths in 2030 can be caused by improper diets.

Association of Diets with Infectious and Parasitic Diseases

Superficially, it seems that infectious and parasitic diseases (contributed 15.76% of the global total DALYs in 2012, the number one contributor, or 11.51% of the global total deaths in 2012) are not associated with daily diets. However, it should be noted that the occurrence of these diseases is largely dependent upon the human body's immunity. The presence of some functional components in diets may improve the human body's immunity whereas that of some toxins may decrease it. Therefore, the occurrence of these diseases is modifiable by immuno-healthy or microorganism inhibiting or improper (for example immuno-depleting) diets.

Association of Diets with Other Diseases

All other causes which contributed to the global total DALYs or deaths in 2012 are modifiable or can be caused by daily diets. Improper daily diets may increase the incidence of these diseases. On the other hand, healthy daily diets may decrease the incidence of these diseases.

Summary

The analyses in the above subsections of this section indicates that more than 90% of causes contributing to the global total DALYs or deaths are modifiable or can be caused by daily diets. Therefore, understanding the association of diets with diseases is very necessary for us to prevent or reduce the global total DALYs or deaths in future.

Brief Explanation of Further Works

Because of vast information about the diets and diseases in the literature, it is very difficult to collect them all in a limited space of a book within a limited time. The selected overview of association of diets with some diseases should be a good choice.

Understanding the causes of diseases is the solid basis of preventing them. For most people, it is believed that the prevention of a disease should be more preferable to its treatment. It is very difficult to recover from some kind of diseases by treatments. Especially, most chronic diseases (for example non-communicable diseases) may not be ever cured once developed. Therefore, "Diets and Diseases: Causes and Prevention" should benefit vast number of people in the world. This would help improve life quality and expectance in future.

References

[1] WHO. Global Health Risks: Mortality and burden of disease attributable to selected major risks. Geneva: World Health Organization press; 2009. ISBN 978 92 4 1563871.

[2] WHO. Global summary estimates, Daly estimates, 2000–2012, Estimates for 2000–2012, Health statistics and information systems. Available from: http://www.who.int/healthinfo/global_burden_disease/estimates/en/index2.html.

[3] WHO. Global summary projections, Mortality 2015 and 2030-Baseline Scenario, Projections of mortality and causes of death, 2015 and 2030, Health statistics and information systems. Available from: http://www.who.int/healthinfo/global_burden_disease/projections/en/.

[4] Wu W, Sun R. Toxicological studies of plant proteins: a review. *J App Toxicol.* 2012; 32(6):377-464.

[5] Wu W, Yang Y. Decontamination of aquatic vegetable leaves by removing trace toxic metals during pickling process with acetic acid solution. *Ecol Food Nutr.* 2011; 50(4):368-374.

[6] WHO. Global summary estimates, Disease and injury regional mortality estimates, 2000–2012, Estimates for 2000–2012, Health statistics and information systems. Available from: http://www.who.int/healthinfo/global_burden_disease/estimates/en/index1.html.

In: Diets and Diseases: Causes and Prevention
Editor: Wenbiao Wu
ISBN: 978-1-63484-580-9

Chapter 1

FUNCTIONAL FOOD

Efstathia Tsakali, Panagiotis Thodis and John Tsaknis*
Department of Food Technology, Technological Educational Institute of Athens,
Agiou Spiridonos, Egaleo, Greece

ABSTRACT

The twenty first century is described by a continuous progress in the field of food science: the discovery of nutrients, the guidelines for a healthy diet and the concept of a balanced diet gave to food development increasing dynamics. First came the power to eliminate malnutrition and later, an attempt to limit the excesses concerning the use of certain substances that are harmful to health. Nutritional sciences are ready to face new challenges, including those associated with the spread of the functional foods concept. A formal identification of functional food category is however quite complex, but in short functional foods may be considered technologically advanced and improved food products. These foods besides being in position to reduce the cost of healthcare from the aging population, could also give a commercial potential in the food industry.

INTRODUCTION

Over the last years scientific research has demonstrated the direct and strong link between the human diet and health. New scientific knowledge and the development of new technologies have led to major changes in life-styles, in the societies of abundance of the occidental, industrialized world. But at the same time new challenges, like the increased costs of health care and increased life expectancy, have appeared [1]. The sciences of nutrition and food technology have to, in addition to maintaining the emphasis on a balanced diet, target to optimum nutrition [2], with the objective of maximizing physiological functions in order to ensure both maximum well-being and health and simultaneously minimize the risk of diseases throughout the life-span [1]. While the better understanding of the interactions between genes

* Corresponding author: Department of Food Technology, Technological Educational Institute of Athens, Agiou Spiridonos, 122 43 Egaleo, Greece. Email: jtsaknis@teiath.gr.

and nutrition is achieved [3], this could match the individual's unique biochemical needs with a tailored selection of nutrient intakes for that individual.

For the life and food sciences the new main target should be not only working towards extending life expectancy but also on improving wellness. On the road to optimized nutrition, which is an ambitious and long-term objective, 'functional food' is, amongst others, a new, interesting and stimulating concept [1].

FUNCTIONAL FOODS: DEFINITIONS AND LEGISLATION

An old belief which now has been considerably evidenced is that basic foods, such as fruits and vegetables, naturally contain chemicals (phytochemicals), which - when consumed in the appropriate quantities – have a protective function and assist in the maintenance of well-being. There are cases that even the same phytochemicals have a preventive and/or therapeutic property against the development of certain diseases. Health professionals are gradually recognizing the role of phytochemicals in health enhancement [4, 5], aided in part by the Nutrition Labeling and Education Act of 1990 (NLEA). The NLEA required nutrition labeling for most foods and allowed disease- or health-related messages on food labels.

The term 'functional food' was first used in Japan, in the 1980s, to indicate a food having a high content of natural metabolites with recognized health benefits such as anticancer, antilipidemic, anticholesterol, antimicrobial, antibacterial, antifungal, antiviral, antihypertensive, anti-inflammatory and antioxidant properties [6]. Over the next years the concept found a great acceptance in western world and in 1999, the European Commission's Concerted Action on Functional Food Science in Europe, defined that: a food product can only be considered as functional if together with the basic nutritional impact it has beneficial effects on one or more functions of the human organism thus either improving the general and physical conditions or/and decreasing the risk of the evolution of diseases. The amount of intake and the form of the functional food should be as normally expected for dietary purposes. Therefore, it should not be in the form of pill or capsule but as a normal food [7]. After years of too many legislative frameworks regulating the approval of products a new regulation on nutrition and health claims made on foods (EC No. 1924/2006), a list of authorized claims was to be published for all member states and nutrient profile will be required for food making health claims. In the late 1990s, instead of 'functional foods,' the term "nutraceutical" (from the words nutrition and pharmaceuticals) was also used, but it was not prevailed. However, it should be reiterated that - as supported by American Dietetic Association (ADA) - all foods may be considered as functional at a specific level. It is important to underline that the term functional should not lead to misunderstandings that foods which do not qualify as "functional" are not safe or hygiene. Obviously all foods can be included in a shape healthy eating. The key again is the amount and the combinations, aka balance.

Under the broad term of functional foods a long list of products could be included which could be further divided in five subcategories. The first one includes foods or ingredients which according to strong scientific proofs have a direct impact on the prevention of diseases. Another group of functional foods are those which are enriched or fortified with one or more ingredients with estimated strong effects on the prevention or dietary treatment of a disease or its clinical symptoms. A third subcategory includes specific foods that are directly related to a reduced risk of appearance of some diseases. There is a limited use of such a claim in a commercial level since it is necessary to present in vitro, in vivo and epidemiology studies to support it and by now the clinical results are limited and sometimes questionable [8]. Foods with a reduced content -due to partly or whole removal- of specific ingredients which are proved harmful, substitute the forth subcategory. These foodstuffs are known as diet or light products. Dietary supplements consist the fifth group of functional foods. These are basically ingredients with important biological properties that can be isolated from their natural source and can be consumed directly or to be added in other foodstuffs in order to modify their properties in a functional way. Finally, it is accepted that functional foods can fit in one or more of these subcategories.

Functional foods or components are often classified as novel. This term cannot be compulsory, since novel foods can stop being innovative with the time while they retain their functionality. According to EC Regulation 258/97 the term novel may be used for foods or ingredients which had not been used for human consumption to countries of the European Union (EU) before 1997. As an independent approach of functional foods, legislation is repeated to include functional components such as: foods or ingredients with a new or intentionally modified original molecular structure, foods or their ingredients consisting of or have been isolated from microorganisms, fungi or algae, foods or their ingredients consisting of or that have been isolated from plants or animals, other than those obtained with the traditional propagating or breeding practices and finally foods or ingredients that have been produced with an innovative process which causes significant changes on their composition or on the structure of their components and may influence their nutritional value, their metabolic ability and the levels of undesirable substances therein [8].

Being clearly positioned as part of nutrition, the functional food concept is, however, quite distinct from other approaches like food supplementation or food fortification, and functional foods are different from nutraceuticals, pharmafoods, vitafoods and 'alicaments,' all terms that are not defined conceptually. Functional foods are food products to be taken as a part of the usual diet in order to have beneficial effects that go beyond what are known as traditional nutritional effects. Moreover, these beneficial effects have to be demonstrated scientifically to justify two specific types of claim: the enhanced function claim or the reduction of disease risk claim [6].

In order to highlight the differences of these different food categories which are often wrongly mentioned as "functional food," some short indicative definitions are given below:

Food for specified health use (FOSHU): In Japan, FOSHU is defined as foods that can enhance consumer's health, and as they have been approved for this reason they may bear a label stating the expected benefits to the consumer's health. This classification, however, is in use only in Japan.

Nutraceutical: Nutraceuticals are products derived from food sources that are purported to provide extra health benefits, in addition to the basic nutritional value found in foods. A nutraceutical can either be marketed as a food or as a drug.

Colorectal Food: Foods that are not decomposed in the stomach, but they reach to colon, mainly in the form of insoluble hydrocarbons, providing essential nutrients in intestine microflora.

Medical foods: Foods with specific characteristics which are consumed under medical supervision in order to prevent a disease. This category includes specific nutrients based on scientific evidence and it is subject to medical assessment. These foods are not sold to healthy consumers and the term is mostly used in US.

CONSUMERS' OPINION ON FUNCTIONAL FOOD

Functional foods gained people acceptance and they now have a greater purchasing power in developed countries. The main benefits to consumer's health are associated with metabolism, antioxidant defense, the immune system, behavioral, spiritual well-being, protection of the cardiac system as well as improving the function of the digestive system. Also, the latest surveys show that functional foods have the potential to enhance significantly the control and weight maintenance as it is rich in fibers and proteins and, thus, enhance the feeling of fullness.

The most common functional foods are those fortified with vitamins and/or minerals such as retinol (vitamin A), tocopherol (vitamin E), folic acid, zinc, iron and calcium. More recently, however, attention has moved to foods fortified with various nutrients such as omega-3 fatty acids, phytosterols and phytochemical substances having antioxidant properties such as carotenoids, phenolic compounds (flavonoids, phenolic acids, catechins, stilbenes, curcumin, etc.), phytoestrogens (isoflavones, lignans) or anticarcinogenic agents such as limonene, allicin, glucosinolates and capsaicinoids. All these substances are able to promote good health, but, if in excess, in some cases, they can result in the opposite effect: vitamins C and E protect cells against damage by free radicals thanks to their antioxidant properties, but, vitamin E excess may increase the risk of bleeding, particularly for adults who are also taking an anticoagulant. Occasionally, adults who utilized very high doses developed muscle weakness, fatigue and nausea [6].

Increased affluence and urbanization are also linked to a lifestyle where daily routine requires less physical activity and there is greater access to foods with higher energy densities. There is a real challenge to balance energy intake and expenditure as more and more people are becoming overweight. In 2008, across the 27 countries of the EU, 59% of adult men and 48% of adult women were either overweight or obese [9]. For much of its history, nutrition science has focused on the role of essential nutrients in preventing deficiencies. However, there is now a need to ensure unaltered levels of key nutrients or functional components in the context of declining energy expenditures. Further, the prevalence of chronic non-communicable diseases such as cardiovascular diseases, high blood pressure and type 2 diabetes has increased, leading to concerns about escalating the costs of healthcare and reduced the quality of life. Modern lifestyles and longer life are also linked to various mental health problems such as depression, poor concentration and the loss of memory.

The food industry has showed a profound interest for food products that meet the consumers' demand for a healthy life style and functional foods have a key role. By definition functional foods are not intended only to satisfy dietary and nutritional human needs but also to assist on the prevention of nutrition-related diseases and increase the physical and mental well-being of their consumers. In 2008, the entire functional foods market was worth over an estimated US$ 80 billion, with the US holding a majority share in the nutraceuticals market (35%), followed by Japan (25%) and with the ever-growing European market, currently estimated at US$ 8 billion. India and China are the two major countries known for their production of traditional functional food products and nutraceuticals, but other South-East Asian countries and Gulf nations are developing potential markets [10].

For a health claim to be truthful and not misleading to consumers, its basis and its wording must be fully consistent with scientific evidences. Guidance for substantiation of claims, the nature of the evidence to be provided and its evaluation, has been developed in several countries over the past two decades. In Europe, the Health Claims regulation (Regulation EC No 1924/2006) recognizes the work of the EC Concerted Actions FUFOSE (Functional Food Science in Europe) and PASSCLAIM (Process for the Scientific Support for Claims on Foods) as valuable projects to be taken into account when assessing health claims.

People consider the healthfulness of foods to be an important factor influencing their overall dietary choices [11, 12]. Nutrition and health claims are used to highlight specific properties of foods that contain (added) beneficial ingredients or are lower in nutrients we should be eating less of. Some also view claims as a legitimate educational tool that will have a positive impact on consumer behavior and nutrition awareness and as such contribute to public health [13]. However, taste [14-18], brand and price [19], the attractiveness of the product [12, 20] and packaging [17] seem to be more important than health claims in influencing purchasing decisions [21].

Various studies have investigated how consumers respond to health claims on food and drink products, addressing attitudes to health claims and the products carrying them, understanding of health claims as well as purchasing intentions for foods with health claims on. Depending on whether and how consumers understand the health claim, they will develop an attitude to the claim, which in turn may affect the attitude to the product bearing the claim. Attitudes may affect purchase intentions and ultimately purchasing behavior. Product variables include the food/drink category, the format and wording of the health claim, the functional ingredients and the benefit claimed, but also taste and sensory attributes of the product. Consumer variables include personal beliefs not related to specific claims and products (e.g., about the usefulness of functional foods in general), personal relevance (e.g., due to health concerns or health problems), familiarity with functional ingredients or products containing them and nutrition knowledge [21]. An example is that health claims are more likely to be perceived more positively when linked to products with an overall positive health image, e.g., yoghurt or bread [20, 22-25]. Whereas people view certain foods as more suitable than others to carry health claims [23], no consistency exists as to the most appropriate product categories. Health claims are not by default transferable across product categories, and naturally occurring combinations of functional ingredients and carrier products seem to be preferred [23, 25-27].

Since the range of functional features is quite big, there is a real risk that the widespread use of fortified foods is often accompanied by promising health benefits that are hard to be noticed in a short time, leading to an increased consumer confusion or distortion of perception and food choice in order to have a proper and balanced diet. Nowadays, many companies that take the consumer's defending role, try to limit this risk by reducing the misinformation in this area, through action to monitor and evaluate the correlation between the beneficial effects which must be declared on the product package and have clear scientific evidences is needed [28].

References

[1] Roberfroid MB. Global view on functional foods: European perspectives. *Brit. J. Nutr.* 2002; 88(2):133-138.

[2] Milner J. Functional foods: the US perspective. *Am. J. Clin. Nutri.* 2000; 71:1654-1659.

[3] Kok J. Functional foods: relevance of genetic susceptibility. Proc. of Forum on: Functional Food. Strasbour Council of Europe Publishers; 1999.

[4] ADA Position of the American Dietetic Association: Phytochemicals and functional foods. *J. Am. Dietary Assoc.* 1995; 95:493-496.

[5] Howard BV, Kritchevsky D. Phytochemicals and cardiovascular disease - A statement for healthcare professionals from the American Heart Association. *Circulation* 1997; 95:2591-2593.

[6] Lavecchia T, Tibuzzi A, Giardi MT. Biosensors for Functional Food Safety and Analysis. In: Giardi MT, Rea G, Berra B. editors. *Bio-Farms for Nutraceuticals: Functional Food and Safety Control by Biosensors.* Landes Bioscience/Springer Science + Business Media, LLC dual imprint; 2010.

[7] Diplock A, Aggett P, Bornet F, Roberfroid M. Scientific concepts of functional foods in Europe-consensus document. *Brit. J. Nutr.* 1999; 81(1):1-27.

[8] Sflomos K. *Food Chemistry with Diet Eleme*nts Volume 1. 2nd ed. Athens; 2010.

[9] International Association for the Study of Obesity (IASO) [Internet]. Overweight and obesity in the EU 27. Available from: http://www.iotf.org/database/documents/v2PDF forwebsiteEU27.pdf.

[10] Vergari F, Tibuzzi A, Basile G. An Overview of the Functional Food Market: From Marketing Issues and Commercial Players to Future Demand from Life in Space. In: Giardi MT, Rea G, Berra B. editors. Bio-Farms for Nutraceuticals: Functional Food and Safety Control by Biosensors. *Landes Bioscience*/Springer Science + Business Media, LLC dual imprint; 2010.

[11] Grunert KG. Food quality and safety: Consumer perception and demand. *Eur. Rev. Agric. Econ.* 2005; 32:369-391.

[12] Krystallis A, Maglaras G, Mamalis S. Motivations and cognitive structures of consumers in their purchasing of functional foods. *Food Qual. Prefer.* 2008; 19:525-538.

[13] Williams P. Consumer understanding and use of health claims for foods. *Nutr. Rev.* 2005; 63:256–264.

[14] Lyly M, Roininen K, Honkapaa K, Poutanen K, Latheenmaki L. Factors influencing consumers' willingness to use beverages and ready-to-eat frozen soups containing oat beta-glucan in Finland, France and Sweden. *Food Qual. Prefer.* 2007; 18:242-255.

[15] Sabbe S, Verbeke W, Deliza R, Matta V, Van Damme P. Effect of a health claim and personal characteristics on consumer acceptance of fruit juices with different concentrations of ac¸aı´ (Euterpe oleracea Mart.). *Appetite.* 2009; 53:84-92.

[16] Miele NA, Di Monaco R, Cavella S, Masi P. Effect of meal accompaniments on the acceptability of a walnut oil enriched mayonnaise with and without a health claim. *Food Qual. Prefer.* 2010; 21:470-477.

[17] Lalor F, Madden C, McKenzie K, Wall PG. Health claims on foodstuffs: A focus group study of consumer attitudes. *J. Funct. Foods.* 2011; 3:56-59.

[18] Vidigal MCTR, Minim VPR, Carvalho NB, Milagres MP, Goncalves ACA. Effect of a health claim on consumer acceptance of exotic Brazilian fruit juices: Ac¸aı´ (Euterpe oleracea Mart.), camucamu (Myrciaria dubia), caja´ (Spondias lutea L.) and umbu (Spondias tuberosa Arruda). *Food Res. Int.* 2011; 44:1988-1996.

[19] Ares G, Gimenez A, Deliza R. Influence of three non-sensory factors on consumer choice of functional yogurts over regular ones. *Food Qual. Prefer.* 2010; 21:361-367.

[20] Siegrist M, Stampfli N, Kastenholz H. Consumers' willingness to buy functional foods. The influence of carrier, benefit and trust. *Appetite.* 2008; 51:526-529.

[21] Wills JM, Storcksdieck genannt Bonsmann S, Kolka M, Grunert KG. Symposium 2: Nutrition and health claims: help or hindrance European consumers and health claims: attitudes, understanding and purchasing behaviour. *P. Nutr. Soc.* 2012; 71:229-236.

[22] van Kleef E, van Trijp HC, Luning P. Functional foods: Health claim-food product compatibility and the impact of health claim framing on consumer evaluation. *Appetite.* 2005; 44:299-308.

[23] Dean M, Shepherd R, Arvola A, Vassallo M, Winkelmann M, Claupein E et al. Consumer perceptions of healthy cereal products and production methods. *J. Cereal Sci.* 2007; 46:188-196.

[24] Kavanagh G, Lalor F, Kennedy, Minogue D, Wall PG. Health psychology and consumers' perception of claims on food. *P. Nutr. Soc.* 2008; 67:E269.

[25] Lähteenmäki L, Lampila P, Grunert KG, Boztug Y, Ueland Ø, Åström A et al. Impact of health-related claims on the perception of other product attributes. *Food Pol.* 2010; 35:230-239.

[26] Teratanavat R, Hooker NH. Consumer valuations and preference heterogeneity for a novel functional food. *J. Food Sci.* 2006; 71:533-541.

[27] Krutulyte R, Grunert KG, Scholderer J, Lähteenmäki L, Hagemann KS, Elgaard P et al. Perceived fit of different combinations of carriers and functional ingredients and its effect on purchase intention. *Food Qual. Prefer.* 2011; 22:11.

In: Diets and Diseases: Causes and Prevention
Editor: Wenbiao Wu
ISBN: 978-1-63484-580-9

Chapter 2

Diets and Cardiovascular Diseases: Impacts of Polyphenols

Jun-ichi Suzuki**, MD, PhD
Department of Advanced Clinical Science and Therapeutics,
The University of Tokyo, Tokyo, Japan

Abstract

Nutritional factors play critical roles in the development of cardiovascular diseases (CVD). There is a strong relationship between the reduction of CVD and the intake of plant-based foods and beverages. However, their effects on human health are still to be elucidated. Polyphenols from tea, coffee, and cacao have received much attention because they are known to have beneficial effects on CVD. The polyphenols in these beverages may reduce the risk of CVD through multiple mechanisms, including anti-oxidant and anti-inflammatory effects. This article reviews the evidence from experimental and clinical studies to show the potential effect of polyphenols from tea, coffee and cacao on the prevention of CVD.

Introduction

It is well known that nutritional factors play critical roles in the etiology of cardiovascular diseases (CVD) [1]. Epidemiological studies have indicated a strong association between the reduction in the incidence of CVD and the consumption of plant-based foods and beverages [2, 3]. Dauchet et al. wrote a review regarding fruits/vegetable consumption and CVD occurrence [4]. This beneficial effect was thought due to the antioxidant properties of vitamins and carotenoids. Recently, many studies showed the significant ability of polyphenols to protect against cellular damages induced by oxidation [5]. However, their

* Corresponding Author Address: Department of Advanced Clinical Science and Therapeutics, The University of Tokyo, 7-3-1 Hongo, Bunkyo, Tokyo 113-8655, Japan; Phone, 81-3-5800-9116; Fax, 81-3-5800-9182. Email: junichisuzuki-circ@umin.ac.jp.

effects on human health are still to be elucidated. To date, polyphenols from coffee, tea and cacao have received much attention because they are known to have beneficial effects on cardiovascular health. The polyphenols in these beverages may reduce the risk of CVD through multiple mechanisms, including anti-oxidant and anti-inflammatory effects. This article reviews the evidence from experimental and clinical studies to show the potential role of coffee, tea and cacao on the prevention of CVD.

EFFECTS OF PHOLYPHENOLS ON CARDIOVASCULAR DISEASE

It is well known that nonalcoholic beverages and fruits contribute to the polyphenols intake [6]. Only a small amount of polyphenol is absorbed and the absorption rate varies depending on the structure of the molecule. Thus, the maximum concentrations in plasma are usually reached between 1 and 6 h after consumption and circulating levels range between 0.1 and 7 μM [7]. Thus, repeated consumption of plant foods is required to sustain the plasma levels of potential bioactive molecules from polyphenols.

Epidemiological studies have revealed the relationship between the extent of polyphenol-rich food consumption and a protective effect on CVD [8-11]. However, some studies showed an inverse association between the consumption of polyphenols and the risk of CVD [12-14]. Thus, the mechanisms of effect of polyphenols on CVD are still to be elucidated. The preventive effect of polyphenols on CVD was attributed to their antioxidant effects [15]. However, substantial results indicate that the direct anti-oxidant action of polyphenols is doubtful [16, 17]. Recently, experts found limited evidence regarding polyphenol-rich products on biomarkers of oxidative stress in humans [18]. According to recent studies, the mechanisms are thought to involve their anti-inflammatory action [19, 20].

TEA CATECHINS

Characteristics of Tea Catechins

Clinical studies indicate potential beneficial effects of tea consumption on CVD risk factors, including endothelial function, lipid profile, and blood pressure. The most consistent findings are for endothelial function. In a meta-analysis, the overall increase in flow-mediated dilatation (FMD) of tea consumption versus placebo was 2.6% of the arterial diameter [21]. Other results from a meta-analysis showed that green tea consumption lowered total and low-density lipoprotein cholesterol concentrations but had no effect on high-density lipoprotein cholesterol [22]. Another meta-analysis showed that tea consumption reduced blood pressure [23].

Furthermore, tea consumption is known to be associated with lower mortality of clinical myocardial infarction [24, 25]. Recently, it was reported that green tea consumption reduced cardiovascular disease mortality in the Japanese population [9]. Catechins are key components of green tea with many biological functions, including anti-inflammatory, anti-oxidative and anti-carcinogenic effects [26-29]. These effects are induced by the suppression of several inflammatory factors including nuclear factor-kappa B (NF-κB), a multipotential promoter of matrix metalloproteinases (MMPs), cytokines and adhesion molecules [30]. The major tea catechins are epigallocathechin-3 gallate (EGCG), epigallocathechin (EGC), epicathechin-3 gallate (ECG) and others. Among them, EGCG has significant anti-inflammatory functions through multiple pathways. It enhanced the functionality of regulatory T cells [31], reduced inflammatory reactions via mitogen-activated protein kinase pathways [32] and inhibited toll-like receptor signaling [33]. EGCG is also known to possess remarkable potential as a chemopreventive agent against prostate [34] and head/neck [35] cancer. EGCG modulates several key molecular signaling pathways at multiple levels and has synergistic or additive effects when combined with many other natural or synthetic compounds. While these characteristics of tea catechins have been well documented [36], their effects on cardiovascular diseases have not been well investigated. Recently, we reported the effects of tea catechins on inflammatory cardiovascular diseases such as myocardial ischemia [37], acute myocarditis [38], and rejection after heart transplantation [39]. In this part, we reviewed these reports and other investigations.

Tea Catechins Suppress Myocardial Ischemia

Myocardial ischemia and ventricular remodeling cause significant damage leading to cardiac death. It is well known that NF-κB related inflammation is enhanced by ischemia and reperfusion of myocardium. Activation of NF-κB induces adhesion molecules, cytokines and MMPs which are involved in myocardial ischemia. Thus, decoy against NF-κB reduced myocardial inflammation induced by ischemia/reperfusion injury [40]. Since proinflammatory factors are key components in the positive feedback loop of inflammation, the inhibition is an effective therapy for myocardial reperfusion injury by preventing inflammation [41-44]. The effects of catechins are induced by the suppression of several inflammatory factors including MMPs induced by NF-κB [30].

To clarify the role of catechins on the ischemic hearts, a rat myocardial ischemia model was produced by ligation of the left anterior descending coronary artery and this was continued for 28 days [37]. We used tea catechin THEA-FLAN 90S (Ito-en Co. Tokyo, Japan). The rats were assigned randomly to two groups in each experimental model. Rats in the catechin treated ischemia group (n=9) were orally supplemented with the tea catechins (20 mg/kg/day) twice a day using the intragastric intubation method. Other rats were supplemented with normal foods and water without the catechins (n=10). After ischemic injury, the non-treated ischemia group showed significant decline of blood pressure compared to non-treated sham-operated group. However, the catechin administration negated the decline of the blood pressure compared to that of non-treated ischemia group on days 14 and 21. Echocardiography demonstrated that the non-treated ischemia group showed significantly impaired left ventricular contraction compared to those of non-treated sham-operated group. However, the catechin treatment significantly improved left ventricular wall motion compared to that of non-treated ischemia group on day 28. Pathologically, the anterior wall of the hearts was completely fibrotic and remaining area showed interstitial fibrosis and cell infiltration. However, catechin treated hearts showed significantly less infarct size, infarct length, left ventricular circumference and left ventricular inner diameter than those in the non-treated ischemia group. Immunohistochemically, increased numbers of CD4, CD8, CD11b, and intercellular adhesion molecule (ICAM)-1 positive infiltrating cells were observed in the non-treated ischemia group, while the catechin administration suppressed the positive-cell numbers significantly. To prove the effect of catechins on NF-κB, we performed a sensitive multi-well colorimetric assay. It showed that increased NF-κB activity was observed in hearts in the non-treated ischemia group. However, this enhanced NF-κB activity was abolished by the catechin treatment. Finally, to reveal the role of MMPs, the infarct region and myocardium were separated under a dissecting microscope and they were used zymography as previously reported. This showed that increased gelatinase (MMP-2 and MMP-9) activity was observed in hearts in the non-treated ischemia group. However, this enhanced gelatinase activity was decreased by catechin administration. In summary of myocardial ischemia, we clearly demonstrated that catechins prevented chronic ventricular remodeling after ischemic injury due to the altered expression of MMPs.

Other investigations indicated that catechins had a significant role in the regulation of MMPs in cardiovascular systems. Cheng showed that EGCG blocked the activation of pro-MMP-2, MMP-2, membrane type (MT) 1-MMP in the cultured vascular smooth muscle cells (SMCs). They demonstrated that EGCG enhanced the expression of tissue inhibitor of metalloproteinase (TIMP)-2; the data from decreased TIMP-2 activity using its siRNA suggested that enhanced TIMP-2 expression was critical for the inhibition of SMC invasion by EGCG [45]. Other investigators also demonstrated how the catechin affected on SMCs [46-49] and ECs [50] via MMP and TIMP regulation. Yamazaki et al. reported that (-)-epicatechin had limited increases in the infarct region in rat myocardial ischemia-reperfusion injury models [51]. Catechins are known to have effects on not only cardiovascular cells but also other organs and cells. Ho et al. demonstrated that EGCG suppressed the invasion of human oral cancer cells via decreased production of MMPs. They used cytotoxicity, invasion, and migration assays to investigate the effects of human oral cancer cells using gelatin zymography and casein zymography. They demonstrated that EGCG showed a dose-dependent inhibitory effect on the invasion and migration of cancer cells in the absence of cytotoxicity with decreased expression of MMP-2 and MMP-9 [52]. Zhen et al. demonstrated that EGCG prevented carbon tetrachloride-induced hepatic fibrosis. In that paper, EGCG attenuated hepatic stellate cell activation as well as MMP-2 activity. It also demonstrated that the concanavalin A-induced activation of secreted MMP-2 was inhibited by EGCG through the influence of membrane type 1-MMP activity [53]. Lee et al. evaluated the effects of EGCG on the extracellular matrix changes induced by UV radiation using artificial skin. They showed that EGCG decreased the level of MMP production and increased TIMP levels [54]. Because it is well known that the extracellular matrix metabolism is tightly controlled by the collagen degrading MMPs and TIMPs, catechin plays a significant role in the tissue remodeling via extracellular matrix metabolism.

Following our publication, there were many investigations which indicated that tea catechins suppressed myocardial ischemia. Potenza et al. showed that EGCG improved endothelial function and insulin sensitivity, reduced blood pressure, and protected against myocardial I/R injury in rats [55]. Song et al. demonstrated that EGCG-treatment significantly reduced myocardial infarction. This anti-infarct effect was totally abrogated by a nonselective K(ATP) channel blocker glibenclamide. Similarly, a selective mitochondrial K(ATP) (mK(ATP)) channel blocker 5-hydroxydecanoate also aborted the anti-infarct effect of EGCG. They concluded that the K(ATP) channels were pivotal in EGCG-induced cardioprotection [56]. Kim et al. also showed that EGCG treatment at an early reperfusion period reduced myocardial infarction and improved cardiodynamics in isolated rat hearts [57].

Regarding the above, tea catechins have multibiological functions against myocardial ischemia and reperfusion injury.

Tea Catechins Suppress Myocarditis

Myocarditis is a serious disease in humans, patients with myocarditis may present with rapidly progressive heart failure, shock, or arrhythmia in its severe form. Although acute myocardial inflammation is an essential etiology for the progression, no effective treatment has been elucidated [58-62]. Experimental autoimmune myocarditis (EAM) is a rat model that is characterized by severe myocardial damages and multinucleated giant cell infiltration. This has been used as a disease model of human acute myocarditis [63-67]. To clarify the effect, we supplemented diet which contained catechins from day 0 to day 21 (n=12) or diets with saline without catechins for controls (n=9) to rats. After the induction of EAM, the catechins significantly reduced the heart weight/body weight ratio compared to that of non-treated EAM controls. Echocardiogram demonstrated the catechins improved the cardiac function compared to the controls. Pathologically, non-treated control EAM animals showed severe myocardial cell infiltration and fibrotic lesions. However, the catechin treatment showed significantly less myocardial cell infiltration and fibrosis areas compared to those in controls. Immunohistochemistry revealed that enhanced expression of CD4, CD8, CD11b, ICAM-1 and NF-κB on infiltrating and arterial endothelial cells was observed in non-treated EAM hearts, while the catechins suppressed the expression. To examine expression of cytokine mRNA in EAM hearts, RNase protection assay was used. TNF-alpha mRNA level was markedly decreased in the catechin treated group compared with that of control group. On the other hand, mRNA levels of Th2 cytokines such as interleukin (IL)-4 and IL-10 in the catechin treated group were markedly enhanced compared with that of control group. We demonstrated that the myocardial cell infiltration, fibrosis, proinflammatory cytokines were enhanced in the EAM progression and the catechins suppressed the development of these changes with altered cytokine expression [38].

Other investigators demonstrated that catechins have a significant role in the regulation of cytokines and chemokines in the cardiovascular system. Ahn et al. showed that EGCG prevented TNF-alpha-mediated monocyte chemotactic protein-1 (MCP-1) production and reduced phosphorylation of Akt (Ser473) in bovine coronary artery endothelial cells. In addition, EGCG attenuated TNF-alpha mediated down-regulation of TNF-alpha receptor 1 (TNFR1), but not TNFR2 [68]. It was also reported that catechin inhibited tumor-specific angiogenesis by regulating the production pro-inflammatory cytokines. The paper showed that catechin administration differentially regulated the elevation of cytokines such as IL-1beta, IL-6, and TNF-alpha [69]. Catechin also effected cytokine expression in other organs Armed et al. found that EGCG inhibited IL-1beta-induced IL-6 production in rheumatoid arthritis synovial fibroblasts by inducing alternative splicing of gp130 mRNA. They concluded that prevented IL-6 synthesis by EGCG with a unique mechanism of sgp130 up-regulation was promising as a potential therapeutic agent for rheumatoid arthritis [70]. Crouvezier et al. investigated the effects of catechins on the production of pro- and anti-inflammatory cytokines by human leukocytes in vitro. EGCG decreased the production of IL-1beta and enhanced the production of IL-10, but had no effect on the production of IL-6 or TNF-alpha [71]. In contrast, EGCG treated murine colitis with a significant reduction of NF-κB and AP-1 activation. However, treatment with EGCG did not reduce plasma cytokine levels in this murine model [72]. Although these effects showed anti-inflammatory properties of the catechins, the catechin effects on cytokines are different among the experimental models and time points.

Tea Catechins Prevent Transplant Rejection

Cardiac transplantation has been established in humans, however acute rejection and graft arterial diseases (GAD) are still problems [73-76]. We have demonstrated that adhesion molecules are key players in the progression of cardiac allograft rejection. To confirm the effects of catechins on rejection, we have used a class II allomismatch combination of the mice to perform cardiac transplantation [77]. Some recipient mice (n=8) were orally supplemented with tea catechins (20 mg/kg/day); the other transplanted mice were supplemented with normal water without the catechins (n=10) for control. Although severe myocardial cell infiltration and fibrosis was observed in nontreated allografts at day 60, tea catechins markedly attenuated myocardial cell infiltration and fibrosis. Immunohistochemically, the enhancement of CD4, CD8, CD11b, ICAM-1, and vascular cell adhesion molecule (VCAM)-1 expression was observed in nontreated allograft myocardium and coronary arteries. However, catechin markedly attenuated the expression of all these factors. RNase protection assay was used to examine the expression of cytokine mRNA in hearts. The levels of Th2 cytokine IL-10 were significantly elevated in the catechin treated group compared with that of non-treated group. We also performed cell proliferation assays to examine the effect of the catechins on antigen-induced T cell proliferation. The cell proliferation was suppressed by the catechins in comparison to that in the control group [39]. In the study, we have demonstrated that tea catechins reduced both myocardial remodeling and GAD formation with the suppression of cell adhesion molecules. Because blockade of cell adhesion molecule resulted in the suppression of rejection and induction of immunological tolerance [78-81], adhesion molecules were critical in transplantation. Therefore, the regulation of adhesion molecules by catechins may be clinically effective for the suppression of transplant rejection.

Other studies indicated that catechins played a large role in the regulation of adhesion molecules in inflammatory cardiovascular diseases. Ludwig et al. investigated the effects of various tea catechins on the cytokine-induced expression of ICAM-1, VCAM-1, and endothelial leukocyte adhesion molecule-1 (E-selectin) in human umbilical vein endothelial cells (HUVECs) using ELISA. EGCG prevented the induction of VCAM-1 expression, whereas EC and EGC had few effects [82]. Chae et al. showed that EGCG inhibited the angiotensin II-induced elevation of VCAM-1 and ICAM-1 in the HUVEC plasma membranes via the inhibition of the p38 MAPK and the ERK1/2 signaling pathways [83]. These significant effects of catechins are not only observed in cardiovascular cells but also other organs and cells. Handa et al. reported that catechins inhibited the expression of adhesion molecules on gastric cancer cells, HUVECs, and polymorphonuclear leukocytes (PMNs) [84]. Chen et al. investigated the effect of catechins on substance P-induced bladder hyperactivity. Two week-catechin pretreatment reduced bladder ICAM-1 expression and ameliorated the hyperactive bladder response [85]. Thus, these papers demonstrated that the anti-cell adhesion molecule activity of catechins was observed as a systemic anti-inflammatory effect.

We have demonstrated that the catechin intake significantly suppresses the expression of inflammatory factors including adhesion molecules, cytokines, and MMPs. These factors are known to be regulated by NF-κB, which is a central factor for the development of inflammatory diseases [86]. We have reported the specific inhibition of NF-κB using a decoy in the myocardial ischemia, myocarditis, and heart transplant rejection [87]. In these studies, the NF-κB decoy suppresses many inflammatory factors including adhesion molecules, cytokines, and MMPs. Although catechins are not the specific inhibitors of NF-κB, they have similar effects on the inhibitors such as an IKK inhibitor [88, 89] and other inflammatory factors.

Other investigations indicated that catechins had a significant role in the regulation of NF-κB. In cardiovascular systems, Aneja et al. reported that EGCG attenuated myocardial ischemia reperfusion injury in rats. This beneficial effect of EGCG was associated with a reduction of NF-κB and activator protein-1 DNA binding [90]. Han et al. showed the inhibitory effects of EGCG on rat aortic SMCs via NF-κB down-modulation. In the study, EGCG treatment resulted in significant inhibition in attachment, proliferation and an appreciable cell cycle arrest at both G0/G1- and G2/M-phases in SMCs. The immunoblot analysis revealed that the constitutive expression of NF-κB/p65 nuclear protein in SMCs was lowered by EGCG in both the cytosol and the nucleus [91]. To clarify the mechanism, several investigations were performed. As Kim et al. demonstrated, EGCG suppressed NF-κB activation and the phosphorylation of p38 MAPK and JNK in human astrocytoma U373MG cells [92]. Mackenzie et al. investigated the capacity of EC in Hodgkin's lymphoma cells. They showed that EC inhibited NF-κB-DNA binding activity; the inhibition was not associated with EC antioxidant activity, with changes in p65 phosphorylation or NF-κB nuclear translocation [93].

It is assumed that catechins are the tea components responsible for these beneficial effects. In black tea, catechin concentrations are significantly lower than in green tea. Jochmann et al. compared green and black tea with regard to the amelioration of endothelial function. In bovine aortic endothelial cells, green and black tea significantly increased endothelial NO synthase activity to the same extent. Similarly, both teas induced comparable endothelial-dependent vasodilation in rat aortic rings. In human subjects, the ingestion of green and black tea led to significant increases in flow-mediated dilation. The increase in flow-mediated dilation was not significantly different between the two tea preparations. They concluded that green and black teas were equally effective in improving endothelial function [94]. Thus, the favorable effect of tea catechins can be obtained from not only green tea but also black tea.

In this part, we summarize the beneficial effects of catechins in cardiovascular diseases focusing on inflammation. Catechins exert cardiovascular protective effects through multiple mechanisms, including not only anti-inflammatory, but also anti-oxidative, anti-hypertensive, anti-proliferative, anti-thrombogenic, and lipid lowering effects [95-99]. Although epidemiological studies have shown a positive correlation between green tea consumption and cardiovascular health, the detailed pathophysiology of catechin effects has not yet been elucidated. Therefore, further investigation is needed to develop a new strategy to suppress clinical inflammatory diseases using catechins or its related compounds.

Coffee Chlorogenic Acids (CGA)

Characteristics of CGA

Coffee is a complex beverage with hundreds of bioactive components with potential adverse or beneficial effects on the cardiovascular system. The most abundant bioactive compounds in coffee are polyphenols, caffeine and others. Coffee polyphenols, notably chlorogenic acid (CGA), are known to possess anti-oxidant and anti-inflammatory activities. European studies showed that moderate coffee drinking reduced cardiovascular risk by 31% relative to no consumption.

However, over consumption of coffee significantly increased the risk [100]. A similar J-curve was also observed in a Finnish study [101]. A study of over 40,000 post-menopausal US women showed the hazard ratio of death attributed to cardiovascular diseases was 0.76 for the consumption of 1–3 cups/day, 0.81 for 4–5 cups/day, and 0.87 for ≥ 6 cups/day [102]. Thus, the moderate consumption of coffee may inhibit inflammation and reduce the risk of cardiovascular and other inflammatory diseases.

Few clinical studies of CGA's influence on cardiovascular diseases have been performed. A study showed that the CGA significantly lowered systolic and diastolic blood pressure compared with the placebo group [103]. Normotensive subjects with reduced vasoreactivity were also administered with CGA. There was a significant decrease in plasma homocysteine compared with the baseline value for the CGA group [104]. These results indicate that CGA may decrease the risk of cardiovascular diseases.

A study showed the effect of CGA on spontaneously hypertensive rats. A single ingestion of CGA reduced blood pressure in the rats, an effect that was blocked by the administration of a nitric oxide synthase inhibitor. When spontaneously hypertensive rats were fed diets containing 0.5% CGA for 8 weeks, the development of hypertension was inhibited compared with the control diet group. Dietary CGA also reduced oxidative stress and improved nitric oxide bioavailability by inhibiting the excessive production of reactive oxygen species in the vasculature, and led to the attenuation of endothelial dysfunction [105]. At a more relevant dose, CGA given to mice at 10 mg/kg body weight activated calcineurin and enhanced macrophage functions in normal mice, a possible cardiac benefit [106].

CGA Suppresses Myocardial Infarction

The mortality rate in patients with coronary arterial diseases, including myocardial infarction (MI), is high [107]. Myocardial necrosis and ventricular remodeling after MI lead to arrhythmia, cardiac rupture and heart failure. Many studies showed that macrophage related inflammatory response increased myocardial necrosis [108, 109]. These inflammatory responses lead to an increase of fibroblasts and collagen synthesis [110-113]. To test the hypothesis that CGA can attenuate chronic ventricular remodeling after myocardial ischemia, we performed an oral administration of CGA into murine myocardial ischemia models. The MI model was produced by the permanent ligation of the left anterior descending coronary artery using an 8-0 suture passed under the arteries. Some MI mice were supplemented orally with CGA (30 mg/kg/day, MI+CGA group) as a CGA-treated MI group, and other MI mice received vehicle (MI+vehicle group) as a vehicle-treated MI group. Sham-operated mice without MI also received vehicle (Sham+vehicle group) as a sham group, and sham-operated mice without MI received CGA (30 mg/kg/day, Sham+CGA group, n=8) as a Sham+CGA group. Just before sacrifice on day 14, we measured blood pressure, heart rate, and echocardiogram. We revealed the vehicle-treated MI group showed significantly impaired left ventricular contraction compared to the sham-operated group. However, the CGA-treated MI group showed significantly improved ventricular contraction compared to the vehicle-treated MI group. Severe myocardial fibrosis with enhanced macrophage infiltration was observed in the vehicle-treated ischemia group. CGA attenuated these fibrotic changes with suppressed macrophage infiltration without systemic adverse effects. We concluded that CGA might effectively suppress chronic ventricular remodeling after myocardial ischemia because it is critically involved in the suppression of macrophage infiltration [114].

CGA Prevents Myocarditis

Myocarditis is another serious myocardial disease. Patients with myocarditis in its severest form may suffer from rapidly progressive heart failure, shock, or arrhythmia [115-120]. In patients with myocarditis, autoimmune disease is considered to be responsible for the pathogenesis [121-123]. Autoimmune myocarditis can be induced in mice or rats by immunization with cardiac myosin. This model revealed that reactive oxygen species (ROS) and inflammation are the key modulators of myocarditis [124-126].

A cell adhesion glycoprotein molecule, intercellular adhesion molecule (ICAM)-1 revealed upregulation of ligand expression by inflammatory cytokines as an important switch to initiate adhesion [127]. It has shown that ICAM-1 associates the pathological process of myocarditis [128, 129]. It was reported that ICAM-1 in myocardial cells plays a critical role in the acute viral myocarditis that investigated using ICAM-1 neutralizing antibody [130]. Recent data also revealed that ICAM-1 is expressed by inflammation and ROS [131]. Therefore, it suggests that ICAM-1 is required for the onset of myocarditis. To investigate the effect of CGA on myocarditis, we used a murine model of experimental autoimmune myocarditis (EAM). Balb/c mice were immunized with cardiac myosin peptides and complete Freund's adjuvant. CGA or vehicle (Cont) was administered orally from day 0 to day 21 (n=6 and 7, respectively) and the animals were sacrificed on day 21. CGA significantly suppressed ICAM-1 expression in the EAM hearts.

The suppressed ICAM-1 tended to reduce myocardial fibrosis compared to control EAM hearts. The findings suggest CGA influences the inhibition of cell adhesion in myocarditis, and may have beneficial effects on the progression of myocarditis [132]. Our findings and previous data suggest that the CGA treatment may have beneficial effects on the progression of myocardial diseases.

Cacao Polyphenols

Characteristics of Cacao Polyphenols

Cacao products (e.g., chocolate, cocoa) are the rich sources of flavonoids which are potent antioxidant and anti-inflammatory compounds. Flavanols in cocoa increase the formation of endothelial nitric oxide which promotes vasodilation and blood pressure reduction [133]. The benefits of cacao products on cardiovascular health have been well examined. The results indicated that cocoa or chocolate intake may reduce blood pressure. A recent data found that cocoa or chocolate interventions significantly reduced fasting insulin concentrations, insulin resistance, and mean arterial pressure as well as improved endothelial function [134].

Plant polyphenols are known to suppress inflammation, oxidative stress, and fibrosis [135]. Cacao beans (Theobroma cacao) are rich in polyphenols such as (-)-epicatechin and their oligomeric procyanidins [136]. Previous studies revealed that cacao polyphenols enhance antioxidative activity [137] and down-regulated T lymphocyte activation (138). A recent study reported that cacao polyphenols inhibit the development of atherosclerosis in apolipoprotein E-deficient mice [139]. However, no study to reveal the effect of cacao polyphenol on myocarditis has been reported. Several studies indicate the adiponectin effect of anti-inflammatory response and plant polyphenols, including procyanidins induced adiponectin gene expression [140, 141]. A recent review also suggests cocoa polyphenols have potential to enhance adiponectin gene expression [142], however, concrete data was not shown.

Cacao Polyphenol Ameliorates Myocarditis

We revealed that the cacao polyphenol ameliorates myocarditis and it is promising dietary supplement to suppress cardiovascular inflammation and oxidative stress. Histological myocarditis heart sections were stained with HE and Mallory. Cardiac myosin sensitization increased cell infiltration and fibrosis area ratio in vehicle treated hearts. However, cacao polyphenol treatment suppressed these exacerbations. Heart weight to body weight ratios increased in the vehicle group, but did not increase in the cacao polyphenol group. Furthermore, we revealed that mRNA expression of IL-1β and IL-6 in the cacao polyphenol group was lower than in the vehicle group. Cell infiltration-related adhesion molecules, E-selectin and VCAM-1 gene expression were also inhibited by cacao polyphenol in cardiac myosin sensitized hearts. Moreover, collagen type 1 mRNA expression was lower in the cacao polyphenol group compared to the vehicle group.

Summary

Recently, supplements containing polyphenols from green tea, coffee, and cacao have gained attention for preventing diseases, however, the verification of these effects is yet to be fully elucidated. In the future, supplements that contain polyphenols may be useful to treat or prevent various cardiovascular diseases and other autoimmune diseases. In conclusion, polyphenols are a promising dietary supplement that could lead to the suppression of cardiovascular inflammation and oxidative stress.

REFERENCES

[1] O'Toole TE, Conklin DJ, Bhatnagar A. Environmental risk factors for heart disease. *Rev Environ Health,* 2008; 23: 167–202.

[2] Dauchet L, Amouyel P, Dallongeville J. Fruit and vegetable consumption and risk of stroke: a meta-analysis of cohort studies. *Neurology,* 2005; 65: 1193–1197.

[3] Hu FB, Willett WC. Optimal diets for prevention of coronary heart disease. *JAMA,* 2002; 288: 2569–2578.

[4] Dauchet L, Amouyel P, Dallongeville J. Fruits, vegetables and coronary heart disease. *Nat Rev Cardiol.* 2009; 6: 599–608.

[5] Collins AR. Assays for oxidative stress and antioxidant status: applications to research into the biological effectiveness of polyphenols. *Am J Clin Nutr.* 2005; 81(1 Suppl.): 261S-267S.

[6] Clifford MN, Brown JE. Dietary flavonoids and health - broadening the perspective. In: Andersen OM, Markham KR, editors. Flavonoids: Chemistry, Biochemistry and Applications. Boca Raton, FL: CRC Press; 2006.

[7] Manach C, Williamson G, Morand C, Scalbert A, Remesy C. Bioavailability and bioefficacy of polyphenols in humans. I. Review of 97 bioavailability studies. *Am J Clin Nutr.* 2005; 81(1 Suppl.): 230S–242S.

[8] Ghosh D, Scheepens A. Vascular action of polyphenols. *Mol Nutr Food Res.* 2009; 53: 322–331.

[9] Kuriyama S, Shimazu T, Ohmori K, Kikuchi N, Nakaya N, Nishino Y, et al. Green tea consumption and mortality due to cardiovascular disease, cancer, and all causes in Japan: the Ohsaki study. *JAMA,* 2006; 296: 1255–1265.

[10] Mink PJ, Scrafford CG, Barraj LM, Harnack L, Hong CP, Nettleton JA, et al. Flavonoid intake and cardiovascular disease mortality: a prospective study in postmenopausal women. *Am J Clin Nutr.* 2007; 85: 895–909.

[11] Szmitko PE, Verma S. Cardiology patient pages. Red wine and your heart. *Circulation,* 2005; 111(2): e10–e11.

[12] Arts IC, Hollman PC. Polyphenols and disease risk in epidemiologic studies. *Am J Clin Nutr.* 2005; 81(1 Suppl.): 317S-325S.

[13] Hollman PC, Geelen A, Kromhout D. Dietary flavonol intake may lower stroke risk in men and women. *J Nutr.* 2010; 140: 600–604.

[14] Mink PJ, Scrafford CG, Barraj LM, Harnack L, Hong CP, Nettleton JA, et al. Flavonoid intake and cardiovascular disease mortality: a prospective study in postmenopausal women. *Am J Clin Nutr.* 2007; 85: 895–909.

[15] Kris-Etherton PM, Keen CL. Evidence that the antioxidant flavonoids in tea and cocoa are beneficial for cardiovascular health. *Curr Opin Lipidol.* 2002; 13: 41–49.

[16] Halliwell B. Are polyphenols antioxidants or pro-oxidants? What do we learn from cell culture and in vivo studies? *Arch Biochem Biophys.* 2008; 476: 107–112.

[17] Mladenka P, Zatloukalova L, Filipsky T, Hrdina R. Cardiovascular effects of flavonoids are not caused only by direct antioxidant activity. *Free Radic Biol Med.* 2010; 49: 963–975.
[18] Hollman PC, Cassidy A, Comte B, Heinonen M, Richelle M, Richling E, et al. The biological relevance of direct antioxidant effects of polyphenols for cardiovascular health in humans is not established. *J Nutr.* 2011; 141: 989S-1009S.
[19] Gonzalez-Gallego J, Garcia-Mediavilla MV, Sanchez-Campos S, Tunon MJ. Fruit polyphenols, immunity and inflammation. *Br J Nutr.* 2010; 104(Suppl. 3): S15-S27.
[20] Gonzalez R, Ballester I, Lopez-Posadas R, Suarez MD, Zarzuelo A, Martinez-Augustin O, et al. Effects of flavonoids and other polyphenols on inflammation. *Crit Rev Food Sci Nutr.* 2011; 51: 331–362.
[21] Ras RT, Zock PL, Draijer R. Tea consumption enhances endothelial- dependent vasodilation; a meta-analysis. *PLoS One,* 2011; 6: e16974.
[22] Zheng XX, Xu YL, Li SH, Liu XX, Hui R, Huang XH. Green tea intake lowers fasting serum total and LDL cholesterol in adults: a meta-analysis of 14 randomized controlled trials. *Am J Clin Nutr.* 2011; 94:601–610.
[23] Hartley L, Flowers N, Holmes J, Clarke A, Stranges S, Hooper L, et al. Green and black tea for the primary prevention of cardiovascular disease. *Cochrane Database Syst Rev.* 2013; 6: CD009934.
[24] Mukamal KJ, Maclure M, Muller JE, Sherwood JB, Mittleman MA. Tea consumption and mortality after acute myocardial infarction. *Circulation,* 2002; 105: 2476-2481.
[25] Arts ICW, Peter Hollman PCH, Feskens EJM, de Mesquita HBB, Kromhout D. Catechin intake might explain the inverse relation between tea consumption and ischemic heart disease: the Zutphen Elderly Study. *Am J Clin Nutr.* 2001; 74: 227-232.
[26] Ishikawa T, Suzukawa M, Ito T, Yoshida H, Ayaori M, Nishiwaki M, et al. Effect of tea flavonoid supplementation on the susceptibility of low-density lipoprotein to oxidative modification. *Am J Clin Nutr.* 1997; 66: 261-6.
[27] Junkun J, Selman SH, Swiercz R, Skrzypczak-Jankun E. Why drinking tea could prevent cancer. *Nature,* 1997; 387: 561.
[28] Beecher GR, Warden BA, Merken H. Analysis of tea polyphenols. *Proc Soc Exp Biol Med.* 1999; 220: 267-70.
[29] Yang CS, Landau JM, Huang MT, Newmark HL. Inhibition of carcinogenesis by dietary polyphenolic compounds. *Annu Rev Nutr.* 2001; 21: 381-406.
[30] Lin YL, Lin JK. (-)-Epigallocatechin-3-gallate blocks the induction of nitric oxide synthase by down-regulating lipopolysaccharide-induced activity of transcription factor nuclear factor-kappaB. *Mol Pharmacol.* 1997; 52: 465-72.
[31] Yun JM, Jialal I, Devaraj S. Effects of epigallocatechin gallate on regulatory T cell number and function in obese v. lean volunteers. *Br J Nutr.* 2010; 103: 1771-7.
[32] Hirao K, Yumoto H, Nakanishi T, Mukai K, Takahashi K, Takegawa D, et al. Tea catechins reduce inflammatory reactions via mitogen-activated protein kinase pathways in toll-like receptor 2 ligand-stimulated dental pulp cells. *Life Sci.* 2010; 86: 654-60.
[33] Byun EH, Omura T, Yamada K, Tachibana H. Green tea polyphenol epigallocatechin-3-gallate inhibits TLR2 signaling induced by peptidoglycan through the polyphenol sensing molecule 67-kDa laminin receptor. *FEBS Lett.* 2011; 585: 814-20.
[34] Siddiqui IA, Adhami VM, Saleem M, Mukhtar H. Beneficial effects of tea and its polyphenols against prostate cancer. *Mol Nutr Food Res.* 2006; 50: 130-43.

[35] Kim JW, Amin AR, Shin DM. Chemoprevention of head and neck cancer with green tea polyphenols. *Cancer Prev Res.* 2010; 3: 900-9.
[36] Benelli R, Vene R, Bisacchi D, Garbisa S, Albini A. Anti-invasive effects of green tea polyphenol epigallocatechin-3-gallate (EGCG), a natural inhibitor of metallo and serine proteases. *Biol Chem.* 2002; 383: 101-5.
[37] Suzuki J, Ogawa M, Maejima Y, Isobe K, Tanaka H, Sagesaka YM, et al. Tea catechins attenuate chronic ventricular remodeling after myocardial ischemia in rats. *J Mol Cell Cardiol.* 2007; 42: 432-440.
[38] Suzuki J, Ogawa M, Futamatsu H, Kosuge H, Sagesaka YM, Isobe M. Tea catechins improve left ventricular dysfunction, suppress myocardial inflammation, fibrosis, and alter cytokine expression in rat autoimmune myocarditis. *Eur J Heart Fail.* 2007; 9: 152-9.
[39] Suzuki J, Ogawa M, Sagesaka YM, Isobe M. Tea catechins attenuate ventricular remodeling and graft arterial diseases in murine cardiac allografts. *Cardiovasc Res.* 2006; 69: 272-9.
[40] Morishita R, Sugimoto T, Aoki M, Kida I, Tomita N, Moriguchi A, et al. In vivo transfection of cis element "decoy" against nuclear factor-kappaB binding site prevents myocardial infarction. *Nat Med.* 1997; 3: 894-899.
[41] Li C, Browder W, Kao RL. Early activation of transcription factor NF-κB during ischemia in perfused rat heart. *Am J Physiol.* 1999; 45: H543–H552.
[42] Li Q, Verma IM. NF-κB regulation in the immune system. *Nat Rev Immunol.* 2002; 2: 725–734.
[43] Chandrasekar B, Freeman GL. Induction of nuclear factor B and activation protein 1 in postischemic myocardium. *FEBS Lett.* 1997; 401: 30–34.
[44] Onai Y, Suzuki J, Kakuta T, Maejima Y, Haraguchi G, Fukasawa H, et al. Inhibition of IkB phosphorylation in cardiomyocytes attenuates myocardial ischemia/reperfusion injury. *Cardiovasc Res.* 2004; 63: 51-59.
[45] Cheng XW, Kuzuya M, Nakamura K, Liu Z, Di Q, Hasegawa, J et al. Mechanisms of the inhibitory effect of epigallocatechin-3-gallate on cultured human vascular smooth muscle cell invasion. *Arterioscler Thromb Vasc Biol.* 2005; 25: 1864-70.
[46] Ivanov V, Roomi MW, Kalinovsky T, Niedzwiecki A, Rath M. Anti-atherogenic effects of a mixture of ascorbic acid, lysine, proline, arginine, cysteine, and green tea phenolics in human aortic smooth muscle cells. *J Cardiovasc Pharmacol.* 2007; 49: 140-5.
[47] El Bedoui J, Oak MH, Anglard P, Schini-Kerth VB. Catechins prevent vascular smooth muscle cell invasion by inhibiting MT1-MMP activity and MMP-2 expression. *Cardiovasc Res.* 2005; 67: 317-25.
[48] Kim CH, Moon SK. Epigallocatechin-3-gallate causes the p21/WAF1-mediated G(1)-phase arrest of cell cycle and inhibits matrix metalloproteinase-9 expression in TNF-alpha-induced vascular smooth muscle cells. *Arch Biochem Biophys.* 2005; 435: 264-72.
[49] Maeda K, Kuzuya M, Cheng XW, Asai T, Kanda S, Tamaya-Mori N, et al. Green tea catechins inhibit the cultured smooth muscle cell invasion through the basement barrier. *Atherosclerosis,* 2003; 166: 23-30.
[50] Singh AK, Seth P, Anthony P, Husain MM, Madhavan S, Mukhtar H, et al. Green tea constituent epigallocatechin-3-gallate inhibits angiogenic differentiation of human endothelial cells. *Arch Biochem Biophys.* 2002; 401: 29-37.

[51] Yamazaki KG, Romero-Perez D, Barraza-Hidalgo M, Cruz M, Rivas M, Cortez-Gomez B, et al. Short- and long-term effects of (-)-epicatechin on myocardial ischemia-reperfusion injury. *Am J Physiol Heart Circ Physiol.* 2008; 295: H761-7.

[52] Ho YC, Yang SF, Peng CY, Chou MY, Chang YC. Epigallocatechin-3-gallate inhibits the invasion of human oral cancer cells and decreases the productions of matrix metalloproteinases and urokinase-plasminogen activator. *J Oral Pathol Med.* 2007; 36: 588-93.

[53] Zhen MC, Wang Q, Huang XH, Cao LQ, Chen XL, Sun KS, et al. Green tea polyphenol epigallocatechin-3-gallate inhibits oxidative damage and preventive effects on carbon tetrachloride-induced hepatic fibrosis. *J Nutr Biochem.* 2007; 18: 795-805.

[54] Lee JH, Chung JH, Cho KH. The effects of epigallocatechin-3-gallate on extracellular matrix metabolism. *J Dermatol Sci. 2005*; 40: 195-204.

[55] Potenza MA, Marasciulo FL, Tarquinio M, Tiravanti E, Colantuono G, Federici A, et al. EGCG, a green tea polyphenol, improves endothelial function and insulin sensitivity, reduces blood pressure, and protects against myocardial I/R injury in SHR. *Am J Physiol Endocrinol Metab.* 2007; 292: E1378-87.

[56] Song DK, Jang Y, Kim JH, Chun KJ, Lee D, Xu Z. Polyphenol (-)-epigallocatechin gallate during ischemia limits infarct size via mitochondrial K(ATP) channel activation in isolated rat hearts. *J Korean Med Sci.* 2010; 25: 380-6.

[57] Kim CJ, Kim JM, Lee SR, Jang YH, Kim JH, Chun KJ. Polyphenol (-)-epigallocatechin gallate targeting myocardial reperfusion limits infarct size and improves cardiac function. *Korean J Anesthesiol.* 2010; 58: 169-75.

[58] Haas GJ. Etiology, evaluation, and management of acute myocarditis. *Cardiol Rev.* 2001; 9: 88-95.

[59] Oakley CM. Myocarditis, pericarditis and other pericardial diseases. *Heart,* 2000; 84: 449-454.

[60] Batra AS, Lewis AB. Acute myocarditis. *Curr Opin Pediatr.* 2001; 13: 234-239.

[61] Zee-Cheng CS, Tsai CC, Palmer DC, Codd JE, Pennington DG, Williams GA. High incidence of myocarditis by endomyocardial biopsy in patients with idiopathic congestive cardiomyopathy. *J Am Coll Cardiol.* 1984; 3: 63-70.

[62] Parrillo JE, Aretz HT, Palacios I, Fallon JT, Block PC. The results of transvenous endomyocardial biopsy can frequently be used to diagnose myocardial diseases in patients with idiopathic heart failure: endomyocardial biopsies in 100 consecutive patients revealed a substantial incidence of myocarditis. *Circulation,* 1984; 69: 93-101.

[63] Kodama M, Matsumoto Y, Fujiwara M, Masani F, Izumi T, Shibata A. A novel experimental model of giant cell myocarditis induced in rats by immunization with cardiac myosin fraction. *Clin Immunol Immunopathol.* 1990; 57: 250-262.

[64] Kodama M, Izumi T. Experimental autoimmune myocarditis. *Acta Med Bio.* 1991; 39: 1-10.

[65] Kitabayashi H, Isobe M, Watanabe N, Suzuki J, Yazaki Y, Sekiguchi M. FTY 720 prevents development of experimental autoimmune myocarditis through reduction of circulating lymphocytes. *J Cardiovasc Pharmacol.* 2000; 35: 410-416.

[66] Yokoseki O, Suzuki J, Kitabayashi H, Watanabe N, Wada Y, Aoki M, et al. cis element decoy against nuclear factor-κB attenuates development of experimental autoimmune myocarditis in rats. *Circ Res.* 2001; 89: 899-906.

[67] Futamatsu H, Suzuki J, Kosuge H, Yokoseki O, Kamada M, Ito H, et al. Attenuation of experimental autoimmune myocarditis by blocking activated T cells through inducible costimulatory molecule pathway. *Cardiovasc Res.* 2003; 59: 95-104.

[68] Ahn HY, Xu Y, Davidge ST. Epigallocatechin-3-O-gallate inhibits TNFalpha-induced monocyte chemotactic protein-1 production from vascular endothelial cells. *Life Sci.* 2008; 82: 964-8.

[69] Guruvayoorappan C, Kuttan G. (+)-Catechin inhibits tumour angiogenesis and regulates the production of nitric oxide and TNF-alpha in LPS-stimulated macrophages. *Innate Immun.* 2008; 14: 160-74.

[70] Ahmed S, Marotte H, Kwan K, Ruth JH, Campbell PL, Rabquer BJ, et al. Epigallocatechin-3-gallate inhibits IL-6 synthesis and suppresses transsignaling by enhancing soluble gp130 production. *Proc Natl Acad Sci USA.* 2008; 105: 14692-7.

[71] Crouvezier S, Powell B, Keir D, Yaqoob P. The effects of phenolic components of tea on the production of pro- and anti-inflammatory cytokines by human leukocytes in vitro. *Cytokine,* 2001; 13: 280-6.

[72] Abboud PA, Hake PW, Burroughs TJ, Odoms K, O'Connor M, Mangeshkar P, et al. Therapeutic effect of epigallocatechin-3-gallate in a mouse model of colitis. *Eur J Pharmacol.* 2008; 579: 411-7.

[73] Stehlik J, Edwards LB, Kucheryavaya AY, Aurora P, Christie JD, Kirk R, et al. The Registry of the International Society for Heart and Lung Transplantation: twenty-seventh official adult heart transplant report--2010. *J Heart Lung Transplant.* 2010; 29: 1089-1103.

[74] Pinney SP, Mancini D. Cardiac allograft vasculopathy: advances in understanding its pathophysiology, prevention, and treatment. *Curr Opin Cardiol.* 2004; 19: 170-6.

[75] Suzuki J, Isobe M, Aikawa M, Kawauchi M, Shiojima I, Kobayashi N, et al. Nonmuscle and smooth muscle myosin heavy chain expression in rejected cardiac allograft. A study in rat and monkey models. *Circulation,* 1996; 96: 1118-24.

[76] Hosenpud JD. Immune mechanism of cardiac allograft vasculopathy: an update. *Transplant Immunol.* 1993; 1237-49.

[77] Suzuki J, Cole SE, Batirel S, Kosuge H, Shimizu K, Isobe M, et al. Tumor necrosis factor receptor -1 and -2 double deficiency reduces graft arterial disease in murine cardiac allografts. *Am J Transplant.* 2003; 3: 968-976.

[78] Isobe M, Yagita H, Okumura K, Ihara A. Specific acceptance of cardiac allograft after treatment with antibodies to ICAM-1 and LFA-1. *Science,* 1992; 255: 1125-1127.

[79] Kosuge H, Suzuki J, Gotoh R, Koga N, Ito H, Isobe M, et al. The induction of immunological tolerance to cardiac allograft by simultaneous blockade of inducible co-stimulator (ICOS) and CTLA4 pathway. *Transplantation,* 2003; 75:1374-1379.

[80] Kosuge H, Suzuki J, Kakuta T, Haraguchi G, Koga N, Futamatsu H, et al. Attenuation of graft arterial disease by manipulation of the LIGHT pathway. *Arterioscler Thromb Vasc Biol.* 2004; 24: 1409-1415.

[81] Koga N, Suzuki J, Kosuge H, Haraguchi G, Onai Y, Futamatsu H, et al. The blockade of the interaction between PD-1 and PD-L1 accelerates graft arterial disease in cardiac allografts. *Arterioscler Thromb Vasc Biol.* 2004; 24: 2057-2062.

[82] Ludwig A, Lorenz M, Grimbo N, Steinle F, Meiners S, Bartsch C, et al. The tea flavonoid epigallocatechin-3-gallate reduces cytokine-induced VCAM-1 expression and

monocyte adhesion to endothelial cells. *Biochem Biophys Res Commun.* 2004; 316: 659-65.

[83] Chae YJ, Kim CH, Ha TS, Hescheler J, Ahn HY, Sachinidis A. Epigallocatechin-3-O-gallate inhibits the angiotensin II-induced adhesion molecule expression in human umbilical vein endothelial cell via inhibition of MAPK pathways. *Cell Physiol Biochem.* 2007; 20: 859-66.

[84] Handa O, Naito Y, Takagi T, Ishikawa T, Ueda M, Matsumoto N, et al. Inhibitory effects of catechins on neutrophil-dependent gastric inflammation. *Redox Rep.* 2002; 7: 324-8.

[85] Chen WC, Hayakawa S, Shimizu K, Chien CT, Lai MK. Catechins prevents substance P-induced hyperactive bladder in rats via the downregulation of ICAM and ROS. *Neurosci Lett.* 2004; 367: 213-7.

[86] Suzuki J, Ogawa M, Izawa A, Sagesaka YM, Isobe M. Dietary consumption of green tea catechins attenuate hyperlipidemia-induced atherosclerosis and systemic organ damage in mice. *Acta Cardiologica* 2005; 60: 271-276.

[87] Suzuki J, Morishita R, Amano J, Kaneda Y, Issobe M. Decoy against nuclear factor-kappa B attenuates myocardial cell infiltration and arterial neointimal formation in murine cardiac allografts. *Gene Ther.* 2000; 7: 1847-1852.

[88] Wakatsuki S, Suzuki J, Ogawa M, Masumura M, Muto S, Shimizu T, et al. A novel IKK inhibitor suppresses heart failure and chronic remodeling after myocardial ischemia via MMP alteration. *Expert Opin Ther Tar.* 2008; 12: 1469-76.

[89] Onai Y, Suzuki J, Maejima Y, Haraguchi G, Muto S, Itai A. Inhibition of NF-kB improves left ventricular remodeling and cardiac dysfunction after myocardial infarction. *Am J Physiol Heart Circ Physiol.* 2007; 291: H530-8.

[90] Aneja R, Hake PW, Burroughs TJ, Denenberg AG, Wong HR, Zingarelli B. Epigallocatechin, a green tea polyphenol, attenuates myocardial ischemia reperfusion injury in rats. *Mol Med.* 2004; 10: 55-62.

[91] Han DW, Lim HR, Baek HS, Lee MH, Lee SJ, Hyon SH, et al. Inhibitory effects of epigallocatechin-3-O-gallate on serum-stimulated rat aortic smooth muscle cells via nuclear factor-kappaB down-modulation. *Biochem Biophys Res Commun.* 2006; 345: 148-55.

[92] Kim SJ, Jeong HJ, Lee KM, Myung NY, An NH, Yang WM, et al. Epigallocatechin-3-gallate suppresses NF-kappaB activation and phosphorylation of p38 MAPK and JNK in human astrocytoma U373MG cells. *J Nutr Biochem.* 2007; 18: 587-96.

[93] Mackenzie GG, Oteiza PI. Modulation of transcription factor NF-kappaB in Hodgkin's lymphoma cell lines: effect of (-)-epicatechin. *Free Radic Res.* 2006; 40: 1086-94.

[94] Jochmann N, Lorenz M, Krosigk A, Martus P, Böhm V, Baumann G, et al. The efficacy of black tea in ameliorating endothelial function is equivalent to that of green tea. *Br J Nutr.* 2008; 99: 863-8.

[95] Babu PV, Liu D. Green tea catechins and cardiovascular health: an update. *Curr Med Chem.* 2008; 15: 1840-50.

[96] Wolfram S. Effects of green tea and EGCG on cardiovascular and metabolic health. *J Am Coll Nutr.* 2007; 26: 373S-388S.

[97] Shenouda SM, Vita JA. Effects of flavonoid-containing beverages and EGCG on endothelial function. *J Am Coll Nutr.* 2007; 26: 366S-372S.

[98] Basu A, Lucas EA. Mechanisms and effects of green tea on cardiovascular health. *Nutr Rev.* 2007; 65: 361-75.

[99] Cabrera C, Artacho R, Giménez R. Beneficial effects of green tea--a review. *J Am Coll Nutr.* 2006; 25: 79-99.

[100] Panagiotakos DB, Pitsavos C, Chrysohoou C Kokkinos P, Toutouzas P, Stefanadis C. The J-shaped effect of coffee consumption on the risk of developing acute coronary syndromes: the CARDIO2000 case–control study. *J Nutr.* 2003; 133: 3228–32.

[101] Happonen P, Voutilainen S, Salonen. JT. Coffee drinking is dose- dependently related to the risk of acute coronary events in middle-aged men. *J Nutr.* 2004; 134: 2381–6.

[102] Andersen LF, Jacobs Jr. DR, Carlsen MH, Blomhoff R. Consumption of coffee is associated with reduced risk of death attributed to inflammatory and cardiovascular diseases in the Iowa Women's Health Study. *Am J Clin Nutr.* 2006; 83: 1039–46.

[103] Watanabe T, Arai Y, Mitsui Y, Kusaura T, Okawa W, Kajihara Y, et al. The blood pressure-lowering effect and safety of chlorogenic acid from green coffee bean extract in essential hypertension. *Clin Exp Hypertens.* 2006; 28: 439–49.

[104] Ochiai R, Jokura H, Suzuki A, Tokimutsu I, Ohishi M, Komai N, et al. Green coffee bean extract improves human vasoreactivity. *Hypertens Res.* 2004; 27: 731–7.

[105] Suzuki A, Yamamoto N, Jokura H, Yamamoto M, Fujii A, Tokimitsu I, et al. Chlorogenic acid attenuates hypertension and improves endothelial function in spontaneously hypertensive rats. *J Hypertens.* 2006; 24: 1065–73.

[106] Wu HZ, Luo J, Yin YX, Wei Q. Effects of chlorogenic acid, an active compound activating calcineurin, purified from Flos Lonicerae on macrophage. *Acta Pharmacol Sin.* 2004; 25: 1685–9.

[107] Velagaleti RS, Pencina MJ, Murabito JM, Wang TJ, Parikh NI, D'Agostino RB, et al. Long-term trends in the incidence of heart failure after myocardial infarction. *Circulation,* 2008; 118: 2057-62.

[108] Onai Y, Suzuki J, Maejima Y, Haraguchi G, Muto S, Itai A, et al. Inhibition of NF-kappaB improves left ventricular remodeling and cardiac dysfunction after myocardial infarction. *Am J Physiol Heart Circ Physiol.* 2007; 292: H530-8.

[109] Brasier AR. The nuclear factor-kappab-interleukin-6 signalling pathway mediating vascular inflammation. *Cardiovasc Res.* 2010; 86: 211-8.

[110] Frangogiannis NG, Smith CW, Entman ML. The inflammatory response in myocardial infarction. *Cardiovasc Res.* 2002; 53: 31-47.

[111] Kempf T, Zarbock A, Vestweber D, Wollert KC. Anti-inflammatory mechanisms and therapeutic opportunities in myocardial infarct healing. *J Mol Med.* 2012; 90: 361-369.

[112] Vilahur G, Juan-Babot O, Pena E, Onate B, Casani L, Badimon L. Molecular and cellular mechanisms involved in cardiac remodeling after acute myocardial infarction. *J Mol Cell Cardiol.* 2011; 50: 522-533.

[113] Vanhoutte D, Schellings M, Pinto Y, Heymans S. Relevance of matrix metalloproteinases and their inhibitors after myocardial infarction: A temporal and spatial window. *Cardiovasc Res.* 2006; 69: 604-613.

[114] Kanno Y, Watanabe R, Zempo H, Ogawa M, Suzuki J, Isobe M. Chlorogenic acid attenuates ventricular remodeling after myocardial infarction in mice. *Int Heart J.* 2013; 54: 176-80.

[115] Zee-Cheng CS, Tsai CC, Palmer DC, Codd JE, Pennington DG, Williams GA. High incidence of myocarditis by endomyocardial biopsy in patients with idiopathic congestive cardiomyopathy. *J Am Coll Cardiol.* 1984; 3: 63-70.
[116] Oakley CM. Myocarditis, pericarditis and other pericardial diseases. *Heart,* 2000; 84: 449-54.
[117] Batra AS, Lewis AB. Acute myocarditis. *Curr Opin Pediatr.* 2001; 13: 234-9.
[118] Haas GJ. Etiology, evaluation, and management of acute myocarditis. *Cardiol Rev.* 2001; 9: 88-95.
[119] Liu PP, Mason JW. Advances in the understanding of myocarditis. *Circulation,* 2001; 104: 1076-82.
[120] Frustaci A, Chimenti C, Calabrese F, Pieroni M, Thiene G, Maseri A. Immunosuppressive therapy for active lymphocytic myocarditis: virological and immunologic profile of responders versus nonresponders. *Circulation,* 2003; 107: 857-63.
[121] Pummerer CL, Luze K, Grassl G, Bachmaier K, Offner F, Burrell SK, et al. Identification of cardiac myosin peptides capable of inducing autoimmune myocarditis in BALB/c mice. *J Clin Invest.* 1996; 97: 2057-62.
[122] Suzuki J, Ogawa M, Futamatsu H, Kosuge H, Sagesaka YM, Isobe M. Tea catechins improve left ventricular dysfunction, suppress myocardial inflammation and fibrosis, and alter cytokine expression in rat autoimmune myocarditis. *Eur J Heart Fail.* 2007; 9: 152-9.
[123] Suzuki J, Ogawa M, Watanabe R, Morishita R, Hirata Y, Nagai R, et al. Autoimmune giant cell myocarditis: clinical characteristics, experimental models and future treatments. *Expert Opin Ther Tar.* 2011; 15: 1163-72.
[124] Ashigaki N, Suzuki J, Ogawa M, Watanabe R, Aoyama N, Kobayashi N, et al. Periodontal bacteria aggravate experimental autoimmune myocarditis in mice. *Am J Physiol Heart Circ Physiol.* 2013; 304: H740-8.
[125] Ellis, C.R.; Di Salvo, T. Myocarditis: basic and clinical aspects. *Cardiol Rev.* 2007; 15: 170-7.
[126] Kishimoto C, Nimata M, Okabe TA, Shioji K. Immunoglobulin treatment ameliorates myocardial injury in experimental autoimmune myocarditis associated with suppression of reactive oxygen species. *Int J Cardiol.* 2013; 167: 140-5.
[127] Long EO. ICAM-1: getting a grip on leukocyte adhesion. *J Immunol.* 2011; 186: 5021-3.
[128] Seko Y, Matsuda H, Kato K, Hashimoto Y, Yagita H, Okumura K, et al. Expression of intercellular adhesion molecule-1 in murine hearts with acute myocarditis caused by coxsackievirus B3. *J Clin Invest.* 1993; 91: 1327-36.
[129] Nakagawa P, Liu Y, Liao TD, Chen X, Gonzalez GE, Bobbitt KR, et al. Treatment with N-acetyl-seryl-aspartyl-lysyl-proline prevents experimental autoimmune myocarditis in rats. *Am J Physiol Heart Circ Physiol.* 2012; 303: H1114-27.
[130] Kim YS, Ahn Y, Hong MH, Joo SY, Kim KH, Sohn IS, et al. Curcumin attenuates inflammatory responses of TNF-alpha-stimulated human endothelial cells. *J Cardiovasc Pharmacol.* 2007; 50: 41-9.
[131] Phalitakul S, Okada M, Hara Y, Yamawaki H. Vaspin prevents TNF-alpha-induced intracellular adhesion molecule-1 via inhibiting reactive oxygen species-dependent NF-

kappaB and PKCtheta activation in cultured rat vascular smooth muscle cells. *Pharmacol Res.* 2011; 64: 493-500.

[132] Zempo H, Suzuki J, Ogawa M, Watanabe R, Tada Y, Takamura C, et al. Chlorogenic acid suppresses a cell adhesion molecule in experimental autoimmune myocarditis in mice. *Immun Endoc Metab Agents Med Chem.* 2013; 13: 232-236.

[133] Ried K, Sullivan TR, Fakler P, Frank OR, Stocks NP. Effect of cocoa on blood pressure. *Cochrane Database Syst Rev.* 2012; 8: CD008893.

[134] Hooper L, Kay C, Abdelhamid A, Kroon PA, Cohn JS, Rimm EB, et al. Effects of chocolate, cocoa, and flavan-3-ols on cardiovascular health: a systematic review and meta-analysis of randomized trials. *Am J Clin Nutr.* 2012; 95: 740–751.

[135] Ginter E, Simko V. Plant polyphenols in prevention of heart disease. *Bratisl Lek Listy.* 2012; 113: 476-480.

[136] Natsume M, Osakabe N, Yamagishi M, Takizawa T, Nakamura T, Miyatake H, et al. Analyses of polyphenols in cacao liquor, cocoa, and chocolate by normal-phase and reversed-phase HPLC. *Biosci Biotechnol Biochem.* 2000; 64: 2581-2587.

[137] Baba S, Osakabe N, Natsume M, Muto Y, Takizawa T, Terao J. Absorption and urinary excretion of (-)-epicatechin after administration of different levels of cocoa powder or (-)-epicatechin in rats. *J Agric Food Chem.* 2001; 49: 6050-6056.

[138] Ramiro E, Franch A, Castellote C, Andres-Lacueva C, Izquierdo-Pulido M, Castell M. Effect of Theobroma cacao flavonoids on immune activation of a lymphoid cell line. *Br J Nutr.* 2005; 93: 859-866.

[139] Natsume M, Baba S. Suppressive effects of cacao polyphenols on the development of atherosclerosis in apolipoprotein E-deficient mice. *Subcell Biochem.* 2014; 77: 189-198.

[140] Qi GM, Jia LX, Li YL, Li HH, Du J. Adiponectin suppresses angiotensin II-induced inflammation and cardiac fibrosis through activation of macrophage autophagy. *Endocrinol.* 2014; en20132011.

[141] Tian C, Ye X, Zhang R, Long J, Ren W, Ding S, et al. Green tea polyphenols reduced fat deposits in high fat-fed rats via erk1/2-PPARgamma-adiponectin pathway. *PLoS ONE,* 2013; 8: e53796.

[142] Ali F, Ismail A, Kersten S. Molecular mechanisms underlying the potential antiobesity-related diseases effect of cocoa polyphenols. *Mol Nutr Food Res.* 2014; 58: 33-48.

In: Diets and Diseases: Causes and Prevention
Editor: Wenbiao Wu

ISBN: 978-1-63484-580-9

Chapter 3

DIETS AND KIDNEY DISEASES

Oluwatoyin Bolanle Oluwole* and Adesioye Temiloluwa
Department of Food Technology, Federal Institute of Industrial Research, Oshodi, Lagos, Nigeria

ABSTRACT

The causes of kidney diseases are highlighted in this chapter, the risk factors, detection of the disease and diet suitable for managing kidney diseases are recommended. Foods that are low in potassium and phosphorus have been found suitable for managing early stages of kidney diseases. Food industries could develop novel food products from indigenous crops widely cultivated in each country that are low in these minerals for people suffering from early stages of kidney diseases.

Keywords: kidney, disease, detection, manage, industry, diet

INTRODUCTION

In this chapter, the function of the kidney as an organ will be discussed. The main content of the chapter includes the causes and warning signs of kidney disease, the consequences of renal failure, dietary management of chronic kidney disease (CKD) and kidney stones, malnutrition in renal disease, vegetarians diet in CKD management and the relationship between exercise and kidney disease.

* Corresponding Author address: Department of Food Technology, Federal Institute of Industrial Research, Oshodi, Lagos, Nigeria. Email: oluwatoyinoluwole575@yahoo.com.

Functions of the Kidney

The kidney functions as an exocrine and endocrine gland. As an exocrine gland it produces urine and removes toxins and excess water from the body. The normal range of certain compounds in the kidney that aids the removal of toxins include; potassium which must be between 3.5-5mmol/l and calcium between 2.2-2.6mmol/l which are the most important ones [1]. Any deviation in potassium level to about 8 mmol/l leads to death while calcium level of about 4 mmol/l result in low morbidity. Other important compounds are the urea which must be within (3.3-6.7mmol/l), phosphate (0.8-1.4mmol/l) and creatinine (45-120umol/l). The hormones regulated by the kidney include, erythropoietin which aids in the production of red blood cells, vitamin D for the maintenance of healthy bones and renin angiotensin which controls blood pressure [1].

Causes of Kidney Diseases

Kidney disease occurs as a result of a group of disorders collectively known as chronic kidney disease. This disease ranges from urine/kidney abnormalities with normal function to severe kidney failure. Most people affected by chronic kidney disease never reach the severe kidney failure which is the end stage renal disease. Diabetes, glomerulonephritis inflammation, hypertension and polycyst are some of the risk factors that can cause kidney disease [1].

Warning Signs of Kidney Diseases

1. High blood pressure
2. The presence of blood and/or protein in the urine
3. Abnormal range of creatinine and Blood Urea Nitrogen (BUN) blood test
4. A glomerular filtration rate (GFR) less than 60
5. Frequency in urinating particularly at night and difficult or painful urination
6. Puffiness around the eyes, swelling of hands and feet [2]

Consequences of Renal Failure

Renal failure results in a buildup of toxins and water in the body, acidosis (which is the excessive amount of acid in blood plasma below the pH ranges of 7.3-7.45) occurs resulting in muscle wasting, anaemia sets in due to lack of red blood cells, bone diseases occur also because the kidney is unable to regulate vitamin D synthesis and the blood pressure becomes poorly controlled. Patients with renal failure experiences fatigue, nausea, loss of appetite, they may feel cold and itchy and this occurs as a result of the buildup of urea and phosphate. However, as the disease progresses fluid overload will occur causing swelling (oedema) of the face, stomach, legs and body generally, there will also be respiratory distress, cardiac failure, renal bone disease and cardiac arrest [2].

Kidney disease often has no symptoms at the early stage and it can go undetected until it reaches the advanced stage. The major risk factors for kidney disease include those suffering from diabetes, hyperlipidaemia, high blood pressure, obese people, smokers, those with a family history of kidney failure and being age 60 or older [1, 3].

However, a simple urine test and blood test can be used to detect the presence of kidney disease. Albumin creatinine ratio (ACR) is the critical parameter in the urine test which estimates the amount of a type of protein albumin that is in the urine while Glomerular Filtration Rate (GFR) determines how well the kidneys are working to remove wastes from the blood. It is however the best way to check kidney function [4]. A value over 90 is good which indicates a normal kidney function- stage 1, within 60-89 indicates a mildly reduce kidney function which should be monitored- stage 2, between 30-50 GFR indicates a moderately reduced kidney function- stage 3, 15-29 GFR indicates a severely reduced kidney function- stage 4 and 14 or less is very severe and ends the stage of renal failure- stage 5. However, from less than 60 GFR for duration of 3 months proper monitoring and dietary modification should be done because this indicates the onset of kidney disease [1, 3, 5].

There is a relationship between chronic kidney disease, diabetes, cardiovascular disease and hypertension and this makes people who suffer from one of any of this disease susceptible to having any of this other diseases. According to the National service framework for renal services, Figure 1 below shows the interaction between these diseases.

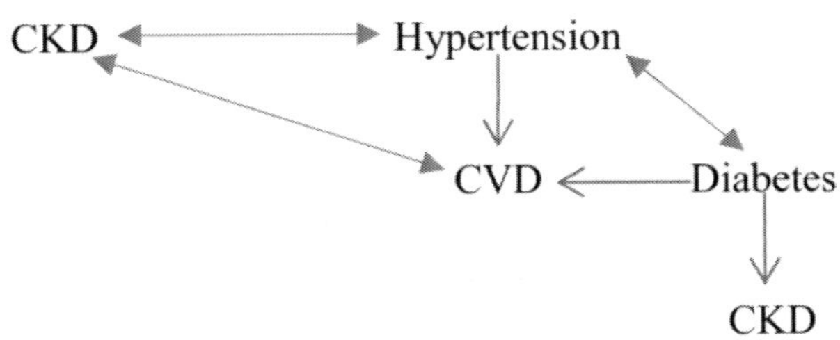

Source: National Service Framework for Renal Services [6].

Figure 1. Interaction of chronic kidney diseases, diabetes, cardiovascular diseases and hypertension.

DIETS AND KIDNEYS

In the occurrence of renal failure the following nutrients should be considered, protein, energy, sodium, phosphate, potassium and fluid. In the early stages of kidney disease one may have little or no limits on what food and drinks. As kidney disease progresses, reduction in phosphorus, potassium, sodium, protein and fluid intake is recommended.

Potassium - It is a mineral found in almost all foods. Potassium is needed in the body to make muscles work when the kidneys are not working well, the potassium level in the body may either be too high or too low. Having too much or too little potassium can cause muscle cramps, breathing difficulty, heart attack, irregular heartbeat and muscle weakness. Foods rich in potassium include fruits and vegetables and in trying to cut down potassium other vitamins are deprived. However, such fruits and vegetables could be boiled to eradicate the potassium but in the same way vitamins are being lost [7]. Food low in potassium includes apples, pineapples, lime, pear, strawberry, tangerines, rasp berry, grapes, white rice, beef, chicken and white bread. Foods with high potassium include banana, oranges, papaya, prunes, brown rice, tomatoes and potatoes [8, 9].

Phosphorus - It is an important mineral found in most foods. It functions well with calcium and vitamin D to maintain healthy bones. Healthy kidneys keep the right balance of phosphorus in the body. When the kidneys are not functioning well, it causes phosphorus to accumulate in the blood. Excessive phosphorus in the blood leads to low calcium in the blood and this causes calcium to be forced out from the bones and these results in weak bones, fracture or osteoporosis has it progresses. High phosphorus in the blood also causes buildup of calcium in the heart, muscles, blood vessels and joints which causes problems like low blood circulation; damage to the heart and other organs and skin ulcers Food low in phosphorus includes corn, rice cereals and unsalted popcorn. Foods high in phosphorus include poultry, beans and nuts [8, 9].

Sodium - It is important for acid-base and water balance in the body. Excess sodium results in water retention in the body called oedema and high blood pressure. Foods rich in sodium include crisps, cottage cheese, gravy mixes, canned tuna and processed meat like bacon, sausages and corned beef. Also salt substitutes should be avoided because most of them contain high potassium chloride which is not good for patients with kidney disease [8].

Protein - Protein is a body building macronutrient important for growth and development. In the case of kidney failure, protein consumption is restricted because in the body metabolism it is broken down into urea which is a waste product that should be eliminated by the kidney however; consuming excessive protein will result to over working of the kidney which will eventually progress into kidney damage [3].

Fluid intake - Excess fluid intake is harmful for patients with kidney failure because of their inability to produce urine frequently which is a form of deposing waste from the body. This results in fluid buildup and affects the normal functioning of the heart and lungs. Therefore, about 1500ml of fluid is recommended for patients with kidney failure at the early stages. Fluid intake includes water, drinks, soups and every food containing liquid and this should all be calculated when measuring fluid intake.

Certain tests such as creatinine, sodium and potassium analysis should be carried out to ascertain the presence of kidney failure, if the values obtained are above the normal expected range steps should be taken to modify dietary intake [10].

Dietary Modification to Kidney Diseases

Dietary modification to kidney diseases include minimizing the progression of the renal failure, maintaining electrolyte levels within safe limits, maintaining or improving fluid balance by restricting fluid intake for instance restriction on beers and red wine. The high potassium present in these beverages is not healthy for patients suffering from renal failure and improving the nutritional status of the patient hereby minimizes health risk factors at all stages [11].

However, changing of dietary intake for renal failure patients reduces both short and long term complications but caution must be put in place to ensure that the diet is well planned and adequately monitored to prevent other risk factors from occurring. Especially, knowing that food is made up of several nutrients and restriction on one nutrient from a particular food may have an impact on other nutrients [10].

At the different stages of CKD, diets must be regulated and monitored closely to minimize risk factors and manage the patient adequately. Stages 1-3 indicate early renal failure and at these stages sodium intake should be modified to about < 100 mmol/d. Likewise buying foods with sodium free labels, low sodium, salt free seasonings and rinsing canned foods such as meats, vegetables and fishes, the DASH (dietary approach to stop hypertension) diets which emphasizes on consuming foods with low salt, low sugar, more fruits and vegetables and less fats could be adopted, energy and lipid must be balanced, and hypertension, hyperlipidaemia, diabetes and obesity must be controlled in patients suffering from them [12]. For instance in diabetes patients, there should be glycaemic control while in controlling lipids the use of statins included and in obese patients gastric banding could be adopted for weight management. Other lifestyle modifications at this stage include moderate alcohol intake, maintaining the ideal BMI or waist circumference, regular exercises and stop smoking. Foods healthy for the heart should be consumed in other to reduce the risk of cardiovascular diseases, fried foods should be avoided instead foods should be boiled, steamed, grilled or toasted, foods such as meats with fat trimmings should be cut off, and healthy vegetable oil should be used for cooking. Foods healthy for the heart include chicken meats without the skin, lean meats, low-fat yoghurt, fishes and vegetables [9].

At stages 4-5, where there is now an established renal failure, minerals and electrolytes balanced must be modified, fluid must be balanced, there must be adequate dietary assessment, and complications arising from cardiovascular diseases, renal bone diseases and malnutrition should be prevented. However to ensure this, regular screening for undernutrition is recommended. Desirably phosphate levels must be within < 1.5-1.7 mmol/l, sodium and potassium must be restricted, and protein intake must be regulated [11]. A dietician is required to advise on protein intake either from animal sources such as meats, fishes, eggs or plant sources such as beans, grains and nuts [10]. In restricting protein intake, foods such as processed meats like ham, sausages, bacon and foods containing added salts like crisps and other canned foods should be avoided. However foods rich in protein healthy for consumption include chicken, lamb, tofu and turkey. Diets and restriction will be determined by the mode of treatment administered. Conservative management of the disease could also be adopted whereby the patient is not placed on dialysis rather the complications are being managed. Medical treatment at this stage includes the use of haemodialysis with drugs and diets, continuous ambulatory peritoneal dialysis (CAPD) with drugs and diets and transplantation. However, some factors may affect getting these treatments and some of these treatments possess certain side effects. For instance, patients with a BMI above 35 will not be considered for transplant, and also there could be a reoccurrence of renal failure from patients suffering from cancer [13].

Nutrition for Patients on Dialysis

Administration of these treatments using the various medical methods requires slightly different nutritional composition in terms of energy, protein, potassium, sodium, phosphorus and fluid. While patients are on dialysis there is a need for increased protein requirement this protein loss occurs as a result of the catabolic effect of dialysis when there is a release of cytokines, acidosis and infection too also affects protein losses.

Energy - Ideally, about 30-35kcal/kg per body weight is required for patients on dialysis. However there food intake could be varied based on individuals but certain factors such as glucose absorption level, activity level and age could affect the attainment of this energy requirement.

Phosphorus - About 85% of the body's phosphorus is present in the bone. Therefore, phosphorus is essential for bone health, nucleic acid structure, energy release and cell membrane structure. For patients on dialysis, phosphorus should be within the range of 1.1-1.7mmol/l compared to 0.9-1.5 mmol/l when not on dialysis. Therefore, proper restriction and monitoring should be ensured by dieticians to prevent vascular calcification and renal bone disease in patients on dialysis. Although phosphorus intake can be restricted to about 600-900mg/day consumption of diet high in protein could increase it to about 1000-1500mg/day hereby exceeding the restriction. This implies that proper nutrient control must be in place to manage patients. Another way to restrict phosphorus absorption is the use of phosphate binders. Phosphate binders aid in controlling phosphorus levels while the right dose is administered at the right time. Foods containing preservatives should be avoided because most preserved foods have a lot of phosphate as preservatives [14].

Potassium - Potassium is essential for acid-base balance and muscle and nerve contraction. The recommended nutrient intake for healthy individuals is 90mmol per day. However, in patients on dialysis there is a restriction on potassium levels to about 50-65 mmol/day. Low and high potassium levels could result in cardiac arrest and therefore for patients with elevated blood levels about 1mmol/kg is recommended. Foods to be restricted include; chocolates, fruits, milk, fruit juice and vegetables. Other factors other than dietary causes could result in high potassium levels including constipation, acidosis, tissue damage and inadequate dialysis/medication [10].

Sodium - The recommended intake is 80-110 mmol/day. Excess sodium intake can lead to thirst which results in increased fluid intake. Foods to be restricted are baked beans, ready-made meals, tinned vegetables, processed foods, ham, salt, cheese, stock cubes and gravies, nuts, salted crisps and tinned fish and meat.

Fluid - Fluid overload promotes cardiac failure, left ventricular hypertrophy, hypertension and respiratory difficulties. Restriction should be on water, alcohol, soft drinks and foods with high fluid content [15].

Malnutrition in Renal Failure

About 20-50% of the population with renal diseases have incidence of malnutrition which is a major cause of morbidity and mortality. Certain factors such as infection, protein losses, hypercatabolism in acidosis, uraemia, depression, anaemia, inadequate dialysis and over restrictive dietary advice all contribute to malnutrition in patients with renal failure [16]. So how do we measure the nutritional status of this people? Several methods such as BMI, blood chemistry, grip strength, anthropometry, food intake and global assessment can be used in measuring the nutritional status of renal patients however, the grip strength and global assessment are the most useful indicators as compared to BMI which is not useful in assessing patients with fluid imbalance, blood chemistry which might be altered as disease progresses, anthropometry which might be inaccurate due to observers error and food intake which may equally be biased due to food choices and disease impairment.

Biochemical measurements such as pre-albumin, albumin, transferrin, retinol binding protein, creatinine, urea, serum electrolytes and total protein could all be assessed to detect malnutrition in renal patients. Prevention of malnutrition is the best treatment however; oral supplementation, intra dialytic parenteral nutrition and nasogastric feeding could be administered. Advice should also be given on food modification to improve their diet [13].

Nutrition after a Kidney Transplant

It is important to know that after a kidney transplant once the new kidney now functions properly there are certain dietary managements that must be adopted. For fluid intake, consumption of plenty of fluid is needed at this stage to prevent dehydration. To hasten the healing process and prevent infection, foods rich in protein such as fish, lean meat, yoghurts, nuts, peas and soy products must be consumed adequately. However foods rich in sodium and potassium should still be restricted to prevent high blood pressure and fluid retention. Other precautions after a kidney transplant include avoiding raw or uncooked foods such as sea foods and meats in order to prevent food-borne illnesses which may arise due to low immune system. Fruits and vegetables should be properly washed before consumption [17].

For weight management, fried foods and high fat/calorie foods should be avoided instead foods high in fibre, nuts, fruits and vegetables should be consumed daily. Regular exercise is essential for weight management, to prevent high blood pressure, to strengthen the heart and to maintain strong bones [18].

Vegetarian Diet in Chronic Kidney Diseases

A vegetarian's diet either a strict vegetarian or a lacto-ovo vegetarian has similar diet restrictions with those on normal diet during CKD management. For protein, high quality protein sources are beneficial for vegetarians such as soy protein which should be included at least daily in every meal. Other sources of high quality protein include tofu, eggs, yoghurt, cooked dry beans and cheese however, yoghurt, cooked dry beans and cheese have high phosphorus and for CKD management phosphorus restriction is important. Therefore, such foods should be consumed minimally and low phosphorus diet should be adopted instead.

Vegetarians consume a lot of fruits and vegetables however, for CKD management potassium must be restricted and high potassium levels can be found in fruits and vegetables such as bananas, apricot, orange, honeydew melon, spinach, tomatoes, sweet potatoes and avocado Therefore, this fruits and vegetables should not be consumed, or consumed minimally or boiled and rinsed before consumption to reduce and remove the potassium present in them. Processed vegetarian foods should not be consumed daily because of high sodium level [19].

EXERCISES AND CHRONIC KIDNEY DISEASES

Lifestyle modification of chronic kidney disease (CKD) patient for physical activity is very important in improving their health. Observing exercise regularly improves the quality of life, improves their sleeping ability, does not cause them any pain, does not affect their appetite negatively and it enhances physical functioning. Regular exercise is important for patients with kidney disease because of certain benefits derived such as regulating weight management thereby preventing obesity, for body fitness and strength, blood pressure control and for diabetes management. Exercises such as swimming and cycling are beneficial especially to reduce cardiovascular complications [20, 21].

DIETS AND KIDNEY STONES

Factors that affect the possibility of having kidney stones include urinary tract infection, fluid intake, diet, gender, age, occupation and metabolic disturbances. Kidney stone is made up of about 80% calcium and oxalate. Factors such as high urine oxalate, calcium, uric acid and sodium, low urine output of less than 2litres per day and low urine magnesium citrates all contribute to the possibility of having calcium oxalates stone formation. Oxalates are waste products made by the body and can also be obtained by consuming foods high in oxalate such as nuts, vegetables like spinach, kale and soy-products. Oxalate is present in most plant food sources because of its ability to dispose excess calcium from plants. Oxalates formation could also be caused by consuming more than 2000mg of vitamin C per day and intestinal over-absorption due to intestinal resection. However, drinking plenty of water about 3litres per day helps in flushing out oxalate therefore this minimizes the occurrence of kidney stone and during hot weather water consumption should increase. Controlling fat intake is important especially for patients with bowel diseases or malabsorption, excess fat binds with calcium alone leaving oxalate which is reabsorbed back into the blood streams. Excess absorption of oxalate thereby combines with calcium in the kidney and this result in calcium oxalate stones [22].

Dietary regulation should therefore be done with caution, while trying to prevent oxalate consumption, fruits and vegetables should not be cut off completely from diets due to its multifunctional benefit in providing various nutrients useful for the body. Soy products such as soy yoghurts, soy nuts, tempeh, soy beverage and tofu should be consumed in moderation because of their high oxalate levels. Calcium intake should not be cut-down except by a dietician's prescription because low calcium intake result in increased oxalate absorption in urine. However, patients suffering from lactose intolerance might have problems with calcium intake because of their inability to consume dairy products but there are other non-dairy food products such as broccoli, lentils, salmons, almonds, bread and foods fortified with calcium such as orange juice and cereals that can be safely consumed by them which will assist in meeting up their daily allowance for calcium. Sodium/salt such as found in canned foods, crisps, bouillon cubes and salt substitutes and animal protein such as found in eggs, meat, fish, livers, scallops and mussels should be consumed minimally; beverages and drinks such as soft drinks, caffeine, alcohol and tea should be restricted; lemon juice should be consumed to increase urine citrate since citrate prevents stones formation in the kidney [22].

CONCLUSION

In chronic kidney disease management, it is important that fluid intake, sodium, potassium, phosphorus and protein intake are well monitored to enhance proper management of the disease. However foods rich in these nutrients should be consumed minimally and physical activity should be encouraged.

REFERENCES

[1] National Kidney Foundation. K/DOQI Clinical Practice Guidelines on Hypertension and Antihypertensive Agents in Chronic Kidney Disease. *Am J Kidney Dis*. 2004; 43(suppl1): S1-290.

[2] Nutrition Education Materials Online. "NEMO," team. *Diet and kidney disease*: A guide for people in the early stages of kidney disease; 2013. Available from: http://www.health.qld.gov.au/masters/copyright.asp.

[3] Martin WF., Armstrong LE, Rodriguez NR. Dietary protein intake and renal function. *Nutr Metab*. 2005; 2:25.

[4] Ash S, Campbell K, MacLaughlin H, McCoy E, Chan M, Anderson K, et al. Evidence based practice guidelines for the nutritional management of chronic kidney disease. *Nutrit Diet*. 2006; 63:S33-S45.

[5] Levey AS., Coresh J, Balk E, Kausz AT., Levin A, Steffes MW. et al. National Kidney Foundation practice guidelines for chronic kidney disease: evaluation, classification, and stratification. *Ann Intern Med*. 2003; 139(2):137-147.

[6] National Service Framework for Renal Services: Part Two: *Chronic Kidney Disease, Acute Renal Failure and End of Life Care*. UK: Department of health; 2005. Available from: http://www.kidney.org.uk/documentlibrary/nsf-pt2.pdf.

[7] Burrowes JD., Ramer NK. Removal of Potassium from Tuberous Root Vegetables by Leaching. *J Ren Nutr*. 2006; 16(4): 304-311.

[8] Chronic Kidney Disease and Nutrition. New Zealand: *Kidney Health*; 2011. Available from: http://www.kidneys.co.nz/resources/file/ckd_&_nutrition.pdf.

[9] NKDEP. *Eating right for kidney health*. NIH Publication No. 14-7405; 2014.

[10] Chan M, Johnson D. *Modification of lifestyle and nutrition interventions for management of early chronic kidney disease*. CARI guidelines. Kidney Health Australia; 2012. Available from: http://www. cari.org.au/CKD/CKD%20early/Modification_of_Llifestyle_Nutrition_ECKD.pdf.

[11] NKDEP. *Chronic Kidney Disease (CKD) and Diet: Assessment, Management and Treatment*. NIH Publication No. 15-7406; 2015.

[12] IOM (Institute of Medicine). *Sodium Intake in Populations: Assessment of Evidence*. Washington, D.C.: National Academy Press; 2013.

[13] Steiber AL., Kopple JD. Vitamin Status and Needs for People with Stages 3-5 Chronic Kidney Disease. *J Ren Nutr*. 2011; 21(5):355-368.

[14] Uribarri J. Phosphorus Homeostasis in Normal Health and in Chronic Kidney Disease Patients with Special Emphasis on Dietary Phosphorus Intake. *Semin Dialys*. 2007; 20(4):295-301.

[15] *Healthy Eating for People on Hemodialysis*. American Kidney Fund; 2010. Available from: http://www.kidneyfund.org/kidney-health/brochures/brochure-pdf/healthy_ eating_for_hemodialysis.pdf.

[16] Krenitsky J. *Nutrition in Renal Failure: Myths and Management*. Practical gastroenterology, Nutrition issues in Gastroenterology series #20; 2004.

[17] UC Davis Medical Center. *Clinical Dietitians, Food and Nutrition Services*. The Regents of the University of California; 2009.

[18] Cloutier M, Adamson E. *The Mediterranean Diet*. New York: Avon Books, Harper Collins Publishers; 2004.

[19] Hogan J. B. *Vegetarian Diets in Chronic Kidney Disease*. Vegetarian Nutrition Dietetic Practice Group; 2010. Available from: http://vegetariannutrition.net/docs/Renal-Vegetarian-Nutrition.pdf.

[20] Kosmadakis GC, Bevington A, Smith AC, Clapp EL, Viana JL, Bishop NC et al. Physical Exercise in Patients with Severe Kidney Disease. *Nephron Clin Pract*. 2010; 115:c7-c16.

[21] Smart NA, Williams AD, Levinger I, Selig S, Howden E, Coombes JS et al. Exercise and Sports Science Australia (ESSA) position statement on exercise and chronic kidney disease. *J Sc Med Sport*. 2013; 16:406-411.

[22] Massey LK, Palmer RG, Horner H. T. Oxalate Content of Soybean Seeds, Soy foods, and other Edible Legumes. *J Agric Food Chem*. 2001; 49(9):4262-6.

In: Diets and Diseases: Causes and Prevention
Editor: Wenbiao Wu
ISBN: 978-1-63484-580-9

Chapter 4

DIETS AND REPRODUCTIVE SYSTEM DISEASE

Omprakash H. Nautiyal*
Professor and Consulting Scientist, Vadodara, Gujarat, India

ABSTRACT

During the menstrual cycle the body tends to crave certain foods, typically fatty, salty and/or sweet. For many, here, the association between diets and the reproductive system comes to stand still. Yet, foods and diets are intricately linked to the reproductive system. What you eat, or fail to eat, can increase or decrease your chances of getting pregnant, worsen your PMS symptoms and possibly even disrupt your menstrual cycle. It is essential to get enough calcium. Women need at least 1,200mg of calcium every day. Some good sources of calcium include low-fat milk, yogurt, broccoli and salmon. If milk is not in the diet, one can increase his calcium intake with soy or rice milk, tofu or kale. One must look for fermented soy products as certain soy products contain phytoestrogens, which can mimic the natural estrogen found in the body, leading to reproductive health difficulties. If there is too much or too little estrogen in one's body, fertility is significantly compromised. Men are different from women in all kinds of ways including their nutritional needs. Just as women need particular nutrients during pregnancy or for protection from breast cancer, men need nutrients that can help them maintain muscle mass, prevent prostate cancer, and more. Many foods that tend to be favorites among men are not the best choices for a good health. They can also enhance performance, from the board room to the bedroom.

Keywords: diet, reproductive disease, nutrition, nutraceutical, antioxidants, vitamins, minerals

*Corresponding Author Address: 102, Shubh Building, Shivalik II, Canal Road, TP 13, Chhani Jakat Naka, Vadodara 390024, Gujarat, India. Email: opnautiyalus@yahoo.com.

INTRODUCTION

It is well known that, during the menstrual cycle, the body tends to crave certain foods, typically fatty, salty and/or sweet. For many, here, the association between diets and the reproductive system comes to stand still. Factually, foods and the diets are intricately linked to the reproductive system. What to eat, or fail to eat, can increase or decrease the chances of getting pregnant, worsen the PMS symptoms and possibly even disrupt menstrual cycle. Every month during ovulation, the pituitary gland in the brain signals the ovaries to produce the hormones oestrogen and progesterone. These hormones help to prepare the uterus in case of a pregnancy. If there is no pregnancy, the hormone levels decrease and menstruation occurs. This increase in hormones helps to explain all the mysterious symptoms of PMS, including craving junk foods and fats [1].

Unfortunately, eating junk foods can actually make one's PMS symptoms worse [2]. Not to mention that one should not give in once in a while. But it is important to make the right food choices, particularly when one has PMS, as eating healthy can help to beat those typical PMS symptoms, like fatigue and bloating. But reaching for the crisps more often than those carrots can do more than worsen PMS. By eating a high-fat diet or starving oneself, one may be putting oneself at risk of developing some serious medical conditions, like amenorrhea (the absence of a period). According to British researchers, if individuals do not eat a healthy, nutritious diet with all the essential vitamins and minerals, their hormones levels can be seriously altered. Some of the theories mention that an imbalanced diet actually causes deficiencies that lead to PMS. Some basic dietary guidelines are mentioned during periods to help control PMS and for better overall health.

It is necessary to ensure one gets enough calcium. Women need at least 1,200mg of calcium every day. Some good sources of calcium include low-fat milk, yogurt, broccoli and salmon.

If milk is not consumed, calcium intake can be increased with soy or rice milk, tofu or kale. Fermented soy products and certain soy products contain phytoestrogens, help to mimic the natural estrogen found in body, leading to reproductive health difficulties. Fertility is significantly compromised if too much or too little estrogen is in the body.

More complex carbohydrates suggested eating whole grain breads, fresh fruits and vegetables when one is hungry.

Keeping hydrated is most essential. Women lose up to 80 mL of blood during a regular period, so it is necessary to keep drinking water to replace body's loss of fluid.

Magnesium (Mg) should be increased in your diets. Foods rich in magnesium, like beans, tofu and peanuts, are meant to reduce bloating in menstruating women. Women should take 200mg per day.

Vitamin E, an antioxidant helps to eliminate some PMS symptoms as well as aiding the circulatory system. Women need 8mg a day. Food with lots of vitamin E includes avocado, egg yolk and liver.

Foods rich in vitamin B_6 which aids in the metabolism of proteins and red blood cells have been cited in numerous studies to relieve depression. Some vitamin B_6 rich foods are potatoes, bananas and oatmeal. An intake of 100mg a day of vitamin B_6 for women is recommended.

It is essential to get vitamin C and zinc. These nutrients support the health of a woman's eggs and reproductive system.

Malnutrition is a major problem in developing countries, and obesity and eating disorders are increasingly common in developing as well as developed countries. The reproductive system is closely linked to nutritional status, especially under-nutrition in the female, and inhibitory pathways involving detectors in the brain suppress ovulation in subjects with weight loss. Recovery may occur after the minimal reacquisition of weight because energy balance is more important than body fat mass. Anorexia nervosa and bulimia nervosa affect up to 5% of women of reproductive age causing amenorrhea, infertility and, in those who do conceive, an increased likelihood of miscarriage. Obesity affects reproduction through fat cell metabolism, steroids and the secretion of proteins such as leptin and adiponectin and through changes induced at the level of important homeostatic factors such as the pancreatic secretion of insulin, androgen synthesis by the production of ovary and sex hormone-binding globulin (SHBG) by the liver.

Adversely, developed nations experience lesser deprivation, but eating disorders and obesity are increasingly common and may be amenable to medical intervention. For females, reproduction involves much greater energy expenditure than for males, and as a protective mechanism against under nutrition, the reproductive axis is closely linked to nutritional status. As one consequence, eating disorders leading to the loss of weight are associated with the reduced frequency or cessation of ovulation. Since energy balance more than absolute weight loss is the key factor, there may be a return of ovulation after no more than a small percentage change in body weight recovery. Obesity, however, is a less reliable risk factor of infertility except among obese women who also have polycystic ovarian disease. This review of nutrition and reproduction will address the clinical conditions that are associated with underweight and overweight in developed countries. It will outline the physiological mechanisms and clinical conditions associated with under nutrition first and then those associated with obesity.

NUTRITION AND FUNCTION OF REPRODUCTIVE SYSTEM

The external environment can have an extreme sensitive influence on the reproductive system. Most animals adjust their pattern of reproduction so that the chances of their offspring surviving are maximal. A common strategy involves the timing of conception by photoperiod and/or rainfall which usually ensures that birth takes place in a season when foods and climatic conditions are favorable, such as spring. Reproduction involves much greater energy expenditure in the female than in the male. The nourishing of the offspring during pregnancy and lactation and their subsequent rearing to adulthood are the biggest expenditure of energy that a female mammal will make in her lifetime. Hence, the female reproductive system is much more sensitive to disruption than the male.

Since reproduction involves energy expenditure, it is sensible that the physiological control mechanisms are linked with appetite and nutrition [3]. Foods are used as a source of energy for a variety of essential and non-essential functions. During deprivation it is necessary to ration available oxidizable substrates in favor of those essential functions involved in staying alive, e.g., keeping warm [4]. Reproduction is dispensable at least in the short term and can be postponed until times are more favorable (Figure1). During lean times animals have devised a number of strategies to reduce energy output such as nestle together in insulated nests (houses), daily torpor or hibernation. Very little energy is detracted to the storage of fats rather calories are mobilized from fat stores in an attempt to maintain energy balance. Thus, it is energy balance not fatness intrinsically that regulates reproductive function.

Under natural conditions, under-nutrition is the dominating factor regulating reproductive activity. In sub-fertility, obesity is an important cause in many modern societies. Adipose tissue is a complex and highly active metabolic and endocrine organ. In addition to adipocytes there are immune cells, connective tissue matrix, nerve tissue and stromovascular cells which together function as an integrated unit. White and brown types of fat tissues differ in composition, appearance and function. White adipose tissue is 60-85% lipid and 90-99% of this lipid is triglyceride. White fatty tissue provides heat regulation, body cushioning and energy storage (triglycerides). Brown fatty tissue derives its color from rich vascularization and densely packed mitochondria. The cells are polygonal in shape, have a considerable volume of cytoplasm and contain multiple lipid droplets of varying size. Their nuclei are round and almost centrally located. Brown fatty tissue may make up 5% of body weight in neonates but disappears by adulthood. It is the site of non-shivering thermo genesis or metabolic heat production without rapid contraction of muscles [5, 6].

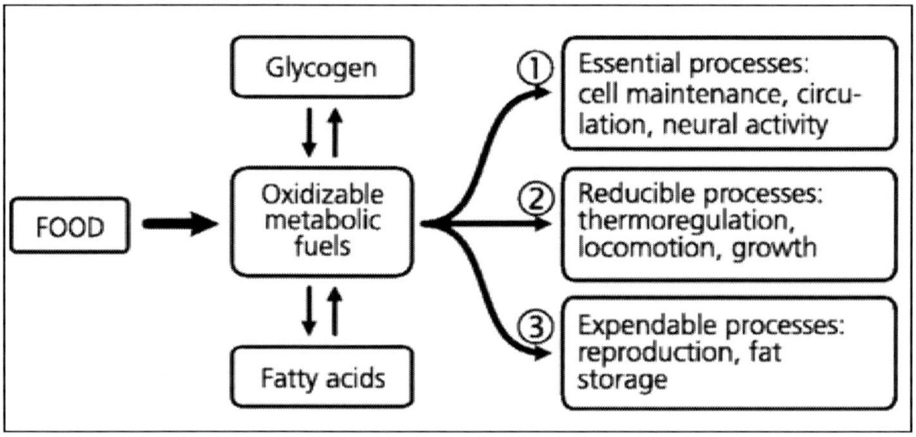

Figure 1. Partitioning of metabolic fats [3].

Benefit of Nutraceuticals Food Supplementation and Antioxidants

Nutritional intake of the long-chain PUFA's Eicosapentaenoic acid (EPA) and DHA is inversely related to sperm concentration and motility, but certainly correlated with the ingestion of the short-chain omega-3 PUFA α-linolenic acid (ALA; 18:3w3). Testicular tissue contains an exceptionally high concentration of the enzymes elongase and desaturase, and mice that were "knocked out" for delta-6-desaturase were infertile with the maturation arrest of spermatogenesis. It seems logical to assume that the long-chain PUFAs cannot pass through the blood-testis barrier, whereas the short chain ALA can do so. The latter is then metabolized into the long-chain PUFAs within the cells of Sertoli thanks to the abundant elongase and desaturase. Therefore, providing an extra amount of ALA to infertile men seems indicated, which is given as linseed- or flaxseed-oil. Vitamin B_6 and zinc better be added, since these are co-factors for the elongase and the desaturase enzymes. Eicosapentaenoid acid and the extract of the bark of the Mediterranean pine tree (Pycnogenol®, Korphag, Geneva, Switzerland) reduce the damage caused by IL-6 to the oocytes and to the Fallopian tubes, through the inhibition of the NF-κB, of the cycloxygenases 1 and 2 (COX 1 and 2), and of the 5-lipoxygenase. Both EPA, given as fish oil, and Pycnogenol® were shown to be beneficial for infertile female patients. The oxidative and anti-oxidant balance can be estimated in blood by measuring the lag-time before extracted LDL-cholesterol is oxidized when exposed to copper. The lag-time was on an average 25% shorter in blood infertile men than in fertile controls, indicating that there was oxidative overload in the former.

Nutraceutical Food Supplements

Normal spermatozoa membrane contains a high concentration of the long chain poly-unsaturated fatty acid (PUFA) of the omega-3 group, docosahexaenoid acid (DHA; 22: 6w3; also called cervonic acid). This procures a high fluidity to the membrane's phospholipids. The cell membrane of poor-quality spermatozoa of patients with varicocele, male accessory gland infection, or idiopathic infertility, contains less DHA, and displays lower fluidity. This is due to inadequate nutritional intake of omega-3 fatty acids, and to higher oxidative load registered among infertile men as compared to fertile controls. Consequently, the capacity of spermatozoa is improved to undergo induced acrosome reaction. The phyto-adaptogen extracted from Lepidium meyenii (MACA) activates the production of the stress suppressing heat-shock protein P70, and can improve fertility in experimental animals. In men Lepidium meyenii was reported to improve sperm quality too (Figure 2) [7].

Cytokinesis and Embryo Development

During the process of cell division cytokinesis inhibits and the contraction of non-muscular myosin II is required for the embryo development. ATP is used by this contractile protein as its energy source, which is produced by the mitochondria. Excess reactive oxygen species in the infertile patients with endometriosis or PID, may reduce the production of ATP, causing inadequate function of the myosin II, and impaired embryo development. Food supplementation during the post-conception weeks with the anti-oxidant Astaxanthin, long-chain PUFA as a source of energy to the mitochondria, carnitines, and the co-enzyme ubiquinone Q10 may improve embryogenesis, cytokenesis, and perhaps implantation. The formulation of the nutraceutical Qualisperm® (Nutriphyt, Oostkamp, Belgium) based on the rationale mentioned above, a novel NFS has been created that is formulated as follows (dose per day): Lepidium meyenii (MACA): 250 mg, Pycnogenol®: 100 mg, L-acetylcarnitine: 100 mg, Carnitine: 100 mg, Co-enzyme ubiquinone Q10: 25mg, Astaxanthin: 8 mg, Zinc-chelate: 7.5 mg, Vitamin B_6 (pyridoxine): 3 mg, Folic acid: 0.2 mg, Vitamin B_{12} (cyanocobalamine): 15 μg. Men should take 2 pills per day together with twice per day 1 g of linseed oil, and women should take 2 pills per day together with 2 g of fish oil, rich in EPA and DHA. Figure 3 shows the association of nutrition with reproduction.

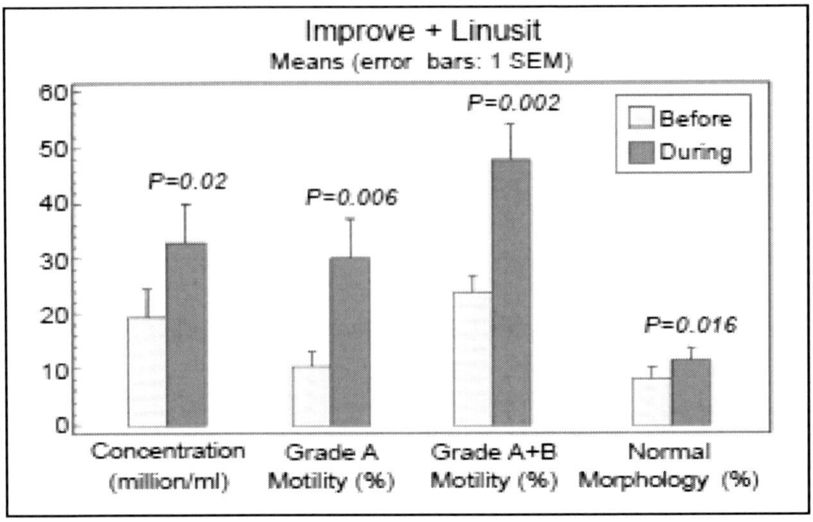

The data are presented as Mean; error bars indicate 1 Standard Error of the Mean. P-Values of statistical significance were calculated using the student's t-test for paired observations [5].

Figure 2. Sperm concentration (in millions per ml of native semen), rapid linear progressive motility (grade A, in %), all progressive motility (grades A and B added, in %), and morphology (% spermatozoa with normal morphological appearance, WHO criteria, Papanicolaou stain), before initiation and after 3 months of intake of the NFS together with linseed oil.

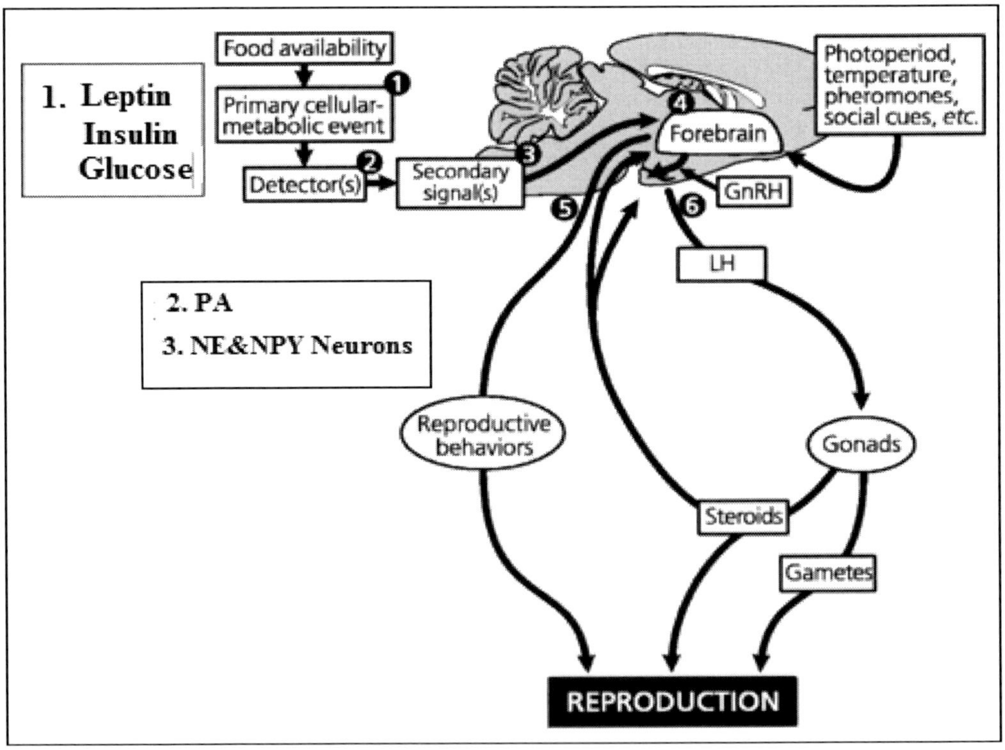

Figure 3. Nutrition and reproduction NE, nor-epinephrine; NPY, neuropeptide Y; PA, postrema [3].

Vitamins and Minerals for a Healthy Reproductive System

The development and proper performance of the reproductive system require the consumption of vitamins, minerals and other nutrients. Nutrition plays a vital role in the development and maturity of the reproductive system through childhood and adolescence. It can even affect the endocrine system which regulates the hormones that rule the functions of the reproductive system. Nutrition can affect fertility and fetal development as well. Striving each day to consume the standard recommended daily intake levels of the vitamins, minerals and other nutrients that the body requires is an important part of the good health and proper functioning of the reproductive system [8].

Hormones are secreted by endocrine glands and hormones are essential to the proper functioning of the reproductive system. Therefore, the wellness of the endocrine gland is a precursor to mature reproductive functioning and health. While several nutrients are directly associated with the production of hormones like manganese which serves to maintain the production of sex hormones many other vitamins and nutrients act as cofactors to a variety of complicated chemical reactions that carry out the tasks for the benefit of the reproductive system [8].

Balanced nutrition is essential in fetal development and folic acid can serve as a way to prevent serious birth defects by reducing the incidences of neural tube defects such as the type that causes spinal bifida. However, this defect occurs so early in fetal development that at the point at which it occurs when the woman has yet to find out that she is actually pregnant. Therefore it is best for any woman of childbearing age to be especially careful to get enough folic acid each day [8].

Vitamin B complex is made up of the vitamins that have a primary role in red blood cell production. The developing fetus receives all nourishments and oxygen via the mother's blood stream. Therefore, making sure to keep red blood cell production up to par is important to the reproductive system, particularly during pregnancy. The nutrients received by the developing fetus will affect every aspect of his or her being [8].

Female Reproductive System Needs

Vitamin B_6 taken twice daily can help to prevent period pains. Also intake of one 50 mg vitamin B complex tablet daily is beneficial.

Magnesium will help with period pains. It should be taken at 200 mg daily. Furthermore, magnesium taken twice per day at 500 mg will help with insomnia, palpitations and period pains.

Evening primrose oil and fish oils both at 500 mg per day can reduce period problems including heavy periods, pain and cramping.

The intake of iron is recommended at 5 mg daily. It should be more if one tends to lose a lot of blood.

Zinc is recommended at 15 mg to help in cases of heavy periods. It is also recommended that Zinc should be taken at 15 mg daily throughout your cycle.

Vitamin A is recommended (as β-carotene). For heavy periods both vitamin A and vitamin B_6 are recommended.

Bioflavonoid can help to balance the hormone levels and regulate the menstrual cycle. It is recommended to take as part of a good vitamin C with bioflavonoids supplement. The intake of vitamin C is recommended to be 500-1000 mg or more daily.

Deficiencies of zinc and vitamin B_6 can result in the absence of periods. An appropriate amount of them should be supplied daily.

Evening primrose oil has been effective in alleviating premenstrual breast tenderness, edema and skin problems. It is recommended to take six to eight 500 mg capsules per day for at least four months. It is best to combine this with a multivitamin and mineral supplement.

Vitamin B complex will help with stress and nervous tension. It should be taken at 50 to 100 mg per day.

Chromium will help if the symptoms are related to blood sugar levels. Sometimes, supplementation of chromium is necessary.

It is generally recommended to limit the intake of sugar, salt, red meat and alcohol. Other recommendations include:

- Eat fish, chicken, whole grains and legumes as the main source of protein;
- Quit smoking;
- Reduce the intake of fats, particularly animal fats, fried foods, and hydrogenated margarines;
- Increase the intake of fiber in the form of fresh fruit and vegetables (particularly leafy green vegetables);
- Eat small amounts regularly, with high quality protein snacks, such as, nuts, seeds, peas and beans, as well as, animal protein, such as, eggs and fish, if sugar or food craving is experienced;
- Take regular outdoor exercise such as walking and swimming;
- Work on managing your stress levels[9].

Pregnancy Related Problems

Many women experience a variety of problems during pregnancy. These discomforts are largely related to hormonal changes in the body or because the body is under additional strain during pregnancy. Common complaints and findings include: anemia, constipation, cramps, varicose veins, vaginal thrush, stretch marks, nausea and vomiting [10].

During pregnancy, some recommendations are as the following:

- Ensure that you get plenty of iron to prevent and treat anemia (see your health professional for dosages);
- Take vitamin C (500 mg per day) with the iron to aid absorption;
- Take at least 400 mcg per day folic acid which is necessary during pregnancy for the healthy development of the fetus.
- Increase fiber intake to help prevent constipation;
- Eat plenty of foods rich in calcium and magnesium to help prevent cramps;
- Take acidophilus for thrush or eat plenty of fresh natural yoghurt.

Vitamin A is linked to growth. Therefore, it is now recommended that all pregnant and breast feeding women take supplements of vitamin A (as beta-carotene) (no more than 10,000 IUs per day) as well as vitamins D and C [10].

Zinc deficiencies during pregnancy are related to low birth weight babies. Therefore, it is recommended that you take 15 mg per day.

Vitamins C and E and bioflavonoids, zinc and brewer's yeast will help to heal damaged vessels causing varicose veins. Furthermore, vitamins E, C and the minerals zinc and silica will help to prevent stretch marks.

Nausea and vomiting during pregnancy will usually respond to iron (5 mg daily), zinc (10 mg daily), magnesium (100 mg daily) and folic acid (200 mcg daily) [10].

Healthy Foods for Women's Reproduction System

In particular certain foods are especially beneficial for women [11] and are only a smaller version of a man's. Female bodies and brains are physically different than male bodies and brains; women are much more sensitive to the artificial hormones and pesticides crammed into many commercial food products, which can wreck havoc on a woman's reproductive system. Protecting your body with antioxidants and other vitamins and nutrients that ward off disease is crucial to keep your system healthy, balanced and functioning at an optimal level. These foods are healthy for all humans to eat but are especially most beneficial for females.

Kale is one of the most potent leafy greens rich in folate, which is an essential B vitamin for women and unborn children; even those females not planning to get pregnant anytime soon should consume it regularly. Kale is also a rich source of calcium (for strong bones) and vitamin C (for immune defense), and B vitamins are known to be mood balancers [11].

Butternut squash and pumpkins as well as orange, root vegetables like sweet potatoes and carrots are rich source of β-carotene which is a powerful antioxidant. B-carotene is known as the protector of vision, but it also protects against breast cancer and repairs damaged skin as well, slowing the signs of aging [11].

Menstruating women must consume iron or they may take the risk of developing anemia; although this important mineral is widely taken in multivitamin form, the body will absorb iron better if foods like spinach, lentils, lean red meat and dark poultry are consumed. If multivitamin are being taken specifically by woman that include iron could result in smooth menstrual [11].

Broccoli is a genuine super food and is a rich source of many vitamins and nutrients. Ounce for ounce, broccoli provides more vitamin C than an orange and also contains the fiber, β -carotene and folic acid. Broccoli is one of the best foods for an expectant mother (or anyone!) who can eat and is particularly useful for those with digestive disorders. Mangoes are extremely good source of vitamin C, a nutrient that fights inflammation and keep the immune system sound. Juicy mangoes are also good source of vitamin A and protect against cervical cancer.

Many women suffer from digestive irregularities such as IBS, and having plenty of natural fiber in the diet from beans, lentils and legumes can help to prevent chronic diseases like colon cancer which kills more women every year than breast cancer. In addition, bulky beans are low in fat, inexpensive and are good aids to beat hunger [11].

Women ought to consume a high quantity of calcium to keep their bones strong against the brittle breaks of osteoporosis. Dairy products are fine sources of calcium, and yogurt gives the added benefit of good bacteria (probiotics) to keep the colon healthy and the whole body system in balance. Premade commercial yogurts are extremely high in sugars and instead must be opted for natural yogurt and flavoring it with honey, or agave syrup and fresh fruits [11].

Figs have been known to contain high levels of vitamin B_6, a nutrient that has been proven to balance the mood and ease the symptoms of PMS. The fiber in figs offers good calories and can sooth many common digestive irregularities as well.

Salmon and other fatty fishes such as mackerel and sardines are rich in omega-3 essential fatty acids, which are indeed necessary for proper brain function as well as protection from arthritis and heart diseases. Most of the people are not aware of these brain-protecting nutrients and must include salmon and other foods high in omega-3 fatty acids several times a week in their daily diets.

Cranberries, strawberries, raspberries, blueberries and black berries are most nutritious and contain powerful anti-cancer agents that play a key role in cell repair and may protect against many forms of diseases, including breast cancer and colon cancer, the two cancers that affect women most. These fruits are vital source of vitamin C, folic acid and antioxidants. Berries safe guard urinary tract infections, help improve vision and may also protect against skin aging [11].

Diets for Male Reproductive System, Lean Proteins

Medicines and surgical methods that can have their own side effects, therefore it is always a better idea to stick to natural remedies especially food and diet cures. By following the routine of a specific diet you can achieve desired outcomes. The list following will help with a perfect diet plan for promoting male reproductive system [11].

One of the nutrients of lean protein should always be included where the male reproductive system is concerned. This supports and strengthens the immune system that will keep away ailments from the reproduction functions as well as promotes the growth and repair of the tissues. Red meats and processed proteins reduce the level of testosterone in the body. One must include the alternatives like Tofu, lentils, beans, white meat skinless, fishes, and dairy products are low in fats. Low fat milk and yoghurt help in proper body functioning [11].

Diets for Male Reproductive System, Selenium Rich Foods

According to researchers, the intakes of foods that are rich in selenium have positive outcomes for the male reproductive system. It activates selenoprotein V that leads to good health of the sperm cells and enhances the reproductive system. Shrimp, Brazil nuts, brown rice and walnuts along with pork, halibut, salmon and chicken are some good sources of selenium. Any of them can be included in the daily diet for best outcomes [11].

Diets for Male Reproductive System, Whole Grains

Including whole grains in the diet will help the reproductive system with the boost of the energy levels on track. The high levels of minerals, vitamins, proteins and fibers in the whole grains will help in reaching the goals [11].

Fresh and seasonal fruits are better and more beneficial as well vegetables including green leafy ones. They are rich in vitamins, fibers, minerals and antioxidants that help the immune system, improve the blood flow as well as enhance the sperm quality and thickness. All these will have a direct impact on the reproductive system. These include all kinds of fruits and vegetables. High levels of potassium in banana have good impact on health management [11].

Diets for Male Reproductive System, Omega Fatty 3 Acids

Omega 3-fatty acids are very potent anti-inflammatory foods, help in many ways and are understood to reduce the levels of triglycerides in the blood. This in turn helps in proper body functioning including the male reproductive system. Some of the best options to be included in the routine diet are flaxseeds, canola oil, eggs, soy, walnuts and fishes like salmon, herring, sardines, mackerel and tuna [12].

Avoidance of Food for Heath Reproductive System

To maintain a healthy reproductive system it is most essential to lead healthy lifestyle that includes healthy diets and regular exercises. Any complications that arise within the reproductive system can lead to damaged reproductive organs and hormonal imbalances, infertility, and pregnancy difficulties. If the health is compromised due to harmful lifestyle choices, the reproductive system will suffer likewise. Therefore, it is important to consume healthful foods and avoid making unhealthy decisions; especially one is planning to become pregnant in near future. In order to keep reproductive system functioning at an optimal level it is strictly suggested not to take the following foods [12].

Caffeine

If woman plans to be pregnant caffeine should not be avoided altogether for a healthy reproductive system; it should be consumed in limited quantities. This is being stimulant and can interfere with fertility if ingested in large amounts. It raises anxiety levels that could further avert the conception process. The consumption of coffee, soda, caffeinated teas and chocolates must be avoided pre and post pregnancy [12].

Sugar

It not only enhances obesity but not even good for the body as it increases the blood sugar and energy levels. For ensuring the best reproductive health one must keep away from the baked foods and junk foods and consume sugars in small quantities. It may also be better to avoid the intake of artificial sweeteners as well.

Alcohol

Alcohol is obviously not good for overall health and, therefore, the reproductive system also suffers due to its consumption. Since alcohol is a depressant it can worsen your mood and disturb PMS symptoms. Above all it can decrease the chances of becoming pregnant and decrease the quality of sperms count. Red wine contains antioxidants so always a good choice instead.

Fast Burning Carbohydrates

White rice, white bread and potatoes are capable of affecting blood sugar levels and can be one of many causes of infertility. On the contrary the reproductive system needs slow digesting carbohydrates that are rich in fibers and whole grains such as brown rice and dark breads can be a good choice.

Processed Foods

In fact *trans*-fats present in many processed foods are not the requirement of the reproductive system and may contribute to infertility. It is always wise to go for natural foods.

Pesticides

Environmental contaminants such as xenoestrogens can cause hormonal imbalances. To prevent these pesticides from harming your reproductive system, fruits and vegetables must be thoroughly washed before consumption. In addition, the source of the drinking water and contaminated chemicals must be up-to-date.

Eating Disorders

Women who are often found to have Amenorrhea (lack of menstrual periods) and oligomenorrhea (infrequent periods) suffer from with anorexia nervosa and bulimia. Reproductive hormones are also reduced in women who maintain a lower-than-normal body weight. An increase in body weight and a balanced food intake will help restore normal reproductive functions.

If there is an eating disorder, the underlying causes of the disorder must be resolved for a permanent recovery. Eating disorders and health problems are associated with each other. The baby can be put at risk for birth defects, low birth weight, or prematurity as well as being born large. So it is best to keep eating habits on track and to ensure ideal body weight before pregnancy. Comprehensive programs involving a psychologist, physician, and dietitian are most helpful. The National Eating Disorders Association and Anorexia Nervosa and Related Eating Disorders are helpful resources [12].

Stress

All stress may not be controlled in life, but one may have more control than one's think. An increase in stress may be due to always saying yes to volunteer projects and in general over scheduling can increase stress. One must take an inventory of their stress and to ensure how one can decrease it or deal with it in a healthful way. It is essential to give a priority to health and stress levels [12].

Oxidative Stress and Antioxidants

Antioxidants play an important role in overall health benefits. Factually, they also play an important role in your fertility. Free radicals can damage the reproductive system and have been correlated with the problems of sperm motility, sperm number, and DNA damage in sperms. Free radicals can affect virtually every step in the reproductive process, from egg maturation to pregnancy. Therefore, an antioxidant-rich diet, like eating expectantly a diet, for parents can improve fertility. Antioxidants include vitamins C and E, folate, carotenoids such as β-carotene and lutein as well as minerals such as selenium, zinc, and copper. Folate and zinc have antioxidant properties that affect both male and female fertility. There are several ways scientists measure foods' antioxidant activity. According to the USDA, a food's antioxidant measurement does not necessarily translate into antioxidant action in the body. The following foods are considered some of the richest in antioxidant contents and be included in the diet "before baby" and beyond.

- *Fruits*: Blackberries, red currants, raspberries, strawberries, blueberries, oranges, pineapple, plums, and pomegranates.
- *Vegetables*: Spinach, Chile peppers, black and green olives, mushrooms, asparagus, arugula, radicchio, beets, broccoli, artichokes, and red peppers
- *Spices*: Clove, allspice, mint, sage, thyme, nutmeg, rosemary, saffron, tarragon, oregano, ginger, cinnamon, natural cocoa.
- *Beverages*: Pomegranate, grape, prune, and cranberry juices (Espresso, coffee, and green and black teas also contain antioxidants but should be consumed in moderation).
- *Nuts, seeds, and grains*: Walnuts, pecans, sunflower seeds, chestnuts, peanuts, pistachios, buckwheat, millet, and barley.

Nutrition and Lifestyle Reign

Nutrition and lifestyle obviously play a critical role in fertility. Nutrition and lifestyle are not only important in the odds of conceiving, but also in carrying a pregnancy to term and having a child who thrives, before going through the expenses and emotional roller coaster of fertility treatments. It is wise for a woman who is trying to conceive to work on improving her diet and that of her partner first. RDs are the perfect source of information for this highly motivated population. It is necessary to remove grains for an optimum nutrition, processed foods, sugars and starches from the diet, and obtain necessary carbohydrates from vegetables, some fruits and starchy sources like sweet potatoes and squash. The healthy fats in the diet especially from sources like coconuts, coconut oil, olives and olive oil, butter, grass-fed meats, eggs, avocado and nuts need to be increased. Proteins especially from grass fed meats, eggs, and nuts are also helpful. There is a need to eat vegetables, especially green leafy varieties and to avoid processed dairy products. Male infertility is a multi-factorial disease process with a number of potential contributing causes. Considering that the majority of male infertility cases are due to deficient sperm production of unknown origin, environmental and nutritional factors must be evaluated. Occupational risk factors, including exposure to heat, chemicals, and heavy metals need to be examined. Lifestyle and dietary choices and pesticide residues may adversely affect fertility. Various nutritional strategies have been presented which have a beneficial impact on egg, female hormone, sperm count, motility, and ultimately on reproduction. It is advisable to consider decreased fertility in both men and women as a physiological early warning system, a "canary in the coal mine," which is acting as a sensitive indicator of environmental disruptions and nutritional imbalances [12].

Essential nutrient deficiencies may adversely affect the functioning of the female reproductive system and cause infertility. Particularly, when deficiencies of folic acid, vitamin B_{12} or iron have been diagnosed and treated, fertility has been restored in women who had been infertile for several years. Conception will not allowed by the body to occur or a pregnancy to continue if it fails to have the basic foundation needed to sustain a pregnancy. Many women turn to a low-fat, high fiber diet in an attempt to increase health and lose weight. Increase in weight loss has been shown to increase fertility, but losing weight in this way may not be effective for increasing fertility because it deprives the body of the necessary proteins and fats necessary for hormone production. The mechanisms involved in this adjustment of reproductive function involve the availability of calories. When Syrian hamsters are administered, 2-de-oxy-D-glucose (DG), which limits glucose oxidation, ovulation cycles are interrupted rapidly. It is likely that this involves both central and peripheral mechanisms. In sheep and rats infusion of DG directly into the lateral ventricles depressed LH secretion. Subsequent experimentation has helped to define the pathway by which calorie deprivation leads to a short-term inhibition of reproductive function. It appears that in the rat the metabolic signals are detected by chemoreceptors in an area of the hind brain area postrema (PA). The signals involved in this are not entirely clear but probably include leptin and insulin/glucose) (Figure 3). Epinephrine, nor-epinephrine and neuropeptide Y (NPY) neurones connect to the forebrain to influence GnRH secretion in the hypothalamus. When the animal is replete, the system is free running. The 'brake' is only applied during the times of negative energy balance and involves NPY neurons [12].

Implications of Treatment with Nutraceuticals Food Supplementation and Mechanisms of Sperm Dysfunction and Female Infertility

High concentration of the long chain poly-unsaturated fatty acid (PUFA) of the omega-3 group, docosahexaenoid acid (DHA; 22: 6w3; also called cervonic acid) is contained within the membrane of normal spermatozoa. This provides a high fluidity to the membrane's phospholipids. Poor-quality spermatozoa cell membrane of patients with varicocele, male accessory gland infection, or idiopathic infertility, contains less DHA, and exhibits lower fluidity. This so happens due to inadequate nutritional intake of omega-3 fatty acids in addition to higher oxidative load registered among infertile men as compared to fertile controls. Consequently, the spermatozoa capacity undergoes induced acrosome reaction. Lepidium meyenii (MACA) extracts containing phyto-adaptogen activate the production of the stress suppressing heat-shock protein P70, and anticipate improving fertility in experimental animals. It has been reported that Lepidium meyenii improves the sperm quality in men (Figure 4).

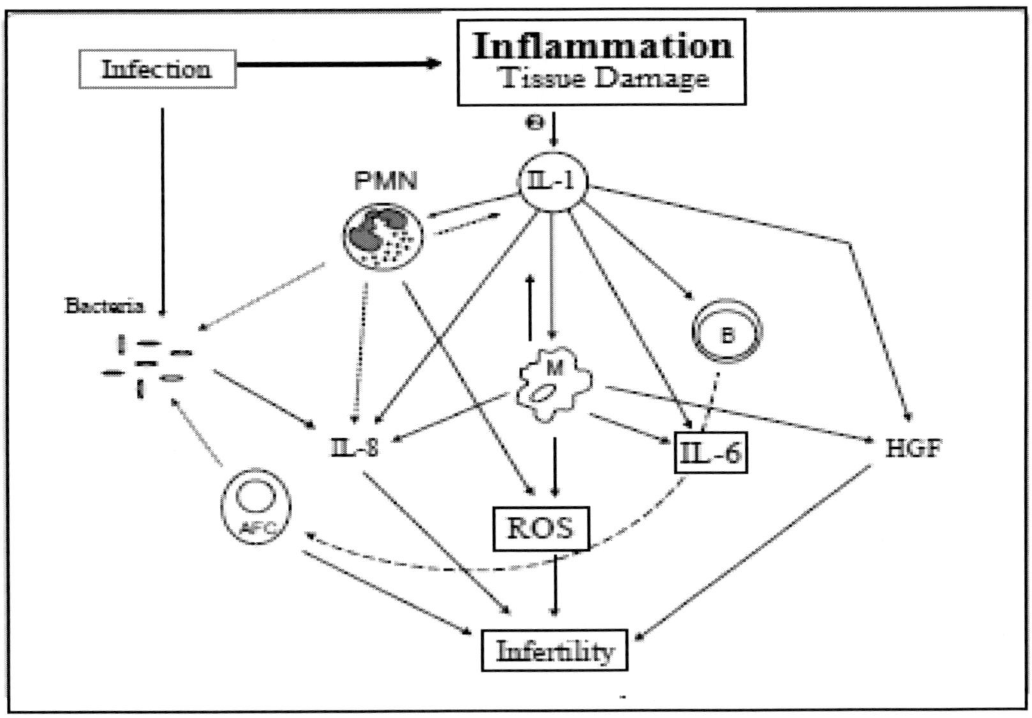

Figure 4. Mechanisms involved in the interaction of infection of the accessory sex glands with male fertility. PMN: polymorphonuclear neutrophilic leukocyte; IL-1: Interleukin 1; IL-6: Interleukin 6; IL-8: Interleukin 8; ROS: reactive oxygen species; HGF: Hepatocyte Growth Factor; M: Monocyte; B: B- lymphocyte; AFC: Antibody Forming Cell [5].

Nutrition and Lifestyle Reign, Prostate Diets

The prostate is a gland present in the male reproductive system, which is of the shape and size of a walnut. Unfortunately, there are many men who suffer from prostate problems, especially an enlarged prostate (also known as Benign Prostate Hyperplasia or BPH), inflammation and prostate cancer. Some of the first signs of prostate problems include problems urinating, traces of blood in the urine and changes in the color of urine. While prostate problems are a lot more common in middle-aged and older men, they can affect just about anybody. It has been seen that men who consume a more calories than is required on a daily basis are a lot more likely to develop prostate problems, as compared to the others. Apart from the intake of excess calories a diet that is very high in animal-based protein could also increase the risks of prostate problems. Caffeine too should be restricted from a healthy prostate diet and therefore soda, coffee, tea and chocolate should be consumed only in limited quantities. Almost all health experts state that it is important for men to follow a healthy prostate diet right from an early age, so that they can avoid prostate problems as they age. The diets that are recommended for various prostate conditions may vary, based on the type of problem, as well as severity of the ailment [13].

Nutrition and Lifestyle Reign, Enlarged Prostate Diets

Most people prefer to treat an enlarged prostate naturally, which includes certain foods. Given below are the nutrients that should be a part of the best prostate diet for an enlarged prostate:

- B-sitosterol, which is found in sugarcane pulp and herbs, such as saw palmetto and pygeum;
- Omega-3 fatty acids, present in flaxseed oil, basil, tuna, salmon oil, halibut and cod liver oil;
- Zinc, generally found in poultry, pork, dairy products, shellfish, eggs, red meat and oysters;
- Vitamin D which can be found in milk green leafy vegetables and liver;
- Vitamin E, present in foods like dry or roast almonds, peanut butter, broccoli, wheat germ oil, sunflower oil and spinach [13].

Nutrition and Lifestyle Reign, Inflamed Prostate Diets

An irritated prostate diet should include foods that contain very high antioxidants, as they enhance the immune system, making it stronger. Some of the foods that should be a part of an irritated or inflamed prostate diet include:

- Watermelons;
- Tomatoes;
- Grapefruit;
- Papaya;
- Red berries;
- Green leafy veggies;
- Red wine;

- Black tea;
- Broccoli;
- Onions;
- Citrus fruit;
- Raspberries.

It is absolutely essential for people to consume a high amount of water for prostate health. There are several prostate dietary supplements also available in the market, which can make up for the lack of adequate nutrients in a diet. However, it is important for people to check with a doctor for daily recommended doses, before adding any supplement to their diet. In fact, men who are elderly or are suffering from any other preexisting medical condition should make sure that they consult a doctor before making any changes to a diet [13].

Nutrition and Lifestyle Reign, Prostate Foods

In order to maintain good prostate health, it is absolutely essential for men to make sure that they eat the healthy prostate foods at all times. There are certain prostate foods to avoid as they could trigger off prostate problems in men. Given below is a list of some of the bad prostate foods, which should be eaten only in limited quantities:

Processed foods are very high in *trans*-fats. This usually includes all commercially prepared food items, such as pastries, pie crusts, canned soup, frozen entrees, fast foods and anything else that may be made using hydrogenated vegetable oil, or even partially hydrogenated vegetable oil. Foods that contain margarine or shortening are also unhealthy for the prostate.

Animal based products, such as cream, butter, dark meat poultry, beef fat, pork, cheese, whole milk, full cream dairy products, beef, poultry with skin and lamb should be avoided, or eaten in limited amounts. It is best to opt for plant based sources of fats, such as olive oil, palm kernel oil, cocoa butter, palm oil and coconut oil.

Refined grains or crabs have been lacking of healthy nutrients like vitamins and fibers during the processing stage. Hence baked goods, polished rice, candies, ice cream, sugar, enriched bread and cereals may not be consumed [14].

Nutrition and Lifestyle Reign, Juice for Prostate

Several men check with health experts about the benefits of juice for prostate problems. Data shows that drinking juice for prostate health can be very effective, as it can treat and prevent major health issues, such as prostate cancer. However, it is important to use the right juice for prostate cancer; commercially prepared juices may not be very effective as they contain high amounts of preservatives and sugar, which reduce their nutritional value. Men should drink homemade fresh juice for prostate improvement [15].

Cranberry juice for prostate is very effective, especially in case of those men who are suffering from prostatitis. It prevents infections, by flushing the bacteria out of the bladder. It also acidifies the urine, so that urethritis and other prostrate problems can be avoided.

Cranberry juice contains anti-cancer properties and therefore, it can prevent prostate cancer [16-18].

Health experts also claim that drinking carrot juice for prostate can be useful, as it can prevent cancer. Another common recommendation from health experts is the consumption of pomegranate juice for prostate cancer. Men also check about the benefits or lime or lemon juice for prostate health. Data shows that taking some amount of lemon or lime juice for prostate can be beneficial, as it boosts immunity and keeps the digestive tract healthy [21, 22].

Table 1. Recommended Dietary Allowance (RDA) for Vitamin A as Preformed Vitamin A (micrograms of Retinol Activity Equivalents [RAE]/day) [19, 20]

Life Stage	Age	Males (mcg/day)	Females (mcg/day)
Infants	0-6 months	400 (AI)	400 (AI)
Infants	7-12 months	500 (AI)	500 (AI)
Children	1-3 years	300	300
Children	4-8 years	400	400
Children	9-13 years	600	600
Adolescents	14-18 years	900	700
Adults	19 years and older	900	700
Pregnancy	18 years and younger	-	750
Pregnancy	19 years and older	-	770
Breast-feeding	18 years and younger	-	1,200
Breast-feeding	19 years and older	-	1,300

Nutrition and Lifestyle Reign, Safety in Pregnancy

Although sufficient vitamin A intake is required for normal fetal development, the consumption of excess vitamin A (such as retinol) during early pregnancy is known to cause birth defects. No increase in the risk of vitamin A-associated birth defects has been observed at doses of preformed vitamin A from supplements below 3,000 mcg RAE/day (10,000 IU/day). Of note, in 2011, the World Health Organization (WHO) recommended vitamin A supplementation (up to 3,000 mcg RAE/day or 7,500 mcg RAE/week) during pregnancy in areas with the high prevalence of vitamin A deficiency for the prevention of blindness. In industrialized countries, pregnant or potentially pregnant women should monitor their intake of vitamin A from fortified foods and foods naturally high in preformed vitamin A (e.g., liver) and avoid taking daily multivitamin supplements that contain more than 1,500 mcg RAE (5,000 IU) of vitamin A. There is no evidence that the consumption of vitamin A from β-carotene might increase the risk of birth defects. The synthetic derivative of retinol, isoretinoin, is known to cause serious birth defects and should not be taken during pregnancy or if there is a possibility of becoming pregnant. T-retinoin (all-*trans*-retinoic acid), another retinol derivative, is prescribed as a topical preparation that is applied to the skin. Although percutaneous absorption of topical T-retinoin is minimal, its use during pregnancy is not recommended. Table 1 reflects data for recommended dietary allowances for vitamin A and retinol activity equivalents per day [21, 22].

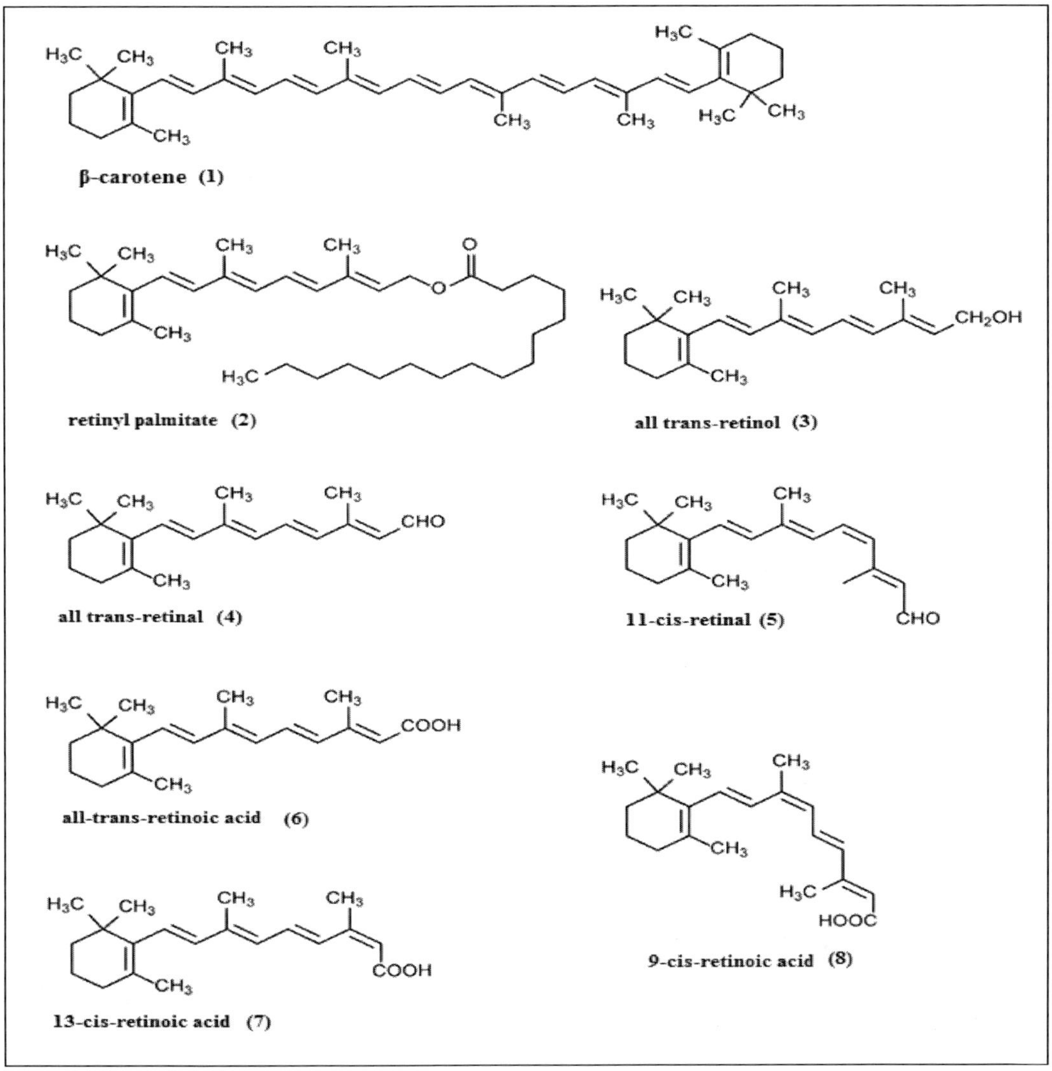

Figure 5. Chemical structures [21, 22].

Vitamin A (Figure 5) is involved in regulating the growth and specialization (differentiation) of virtually all cells in the human body. Vitamin A has important roles in embryonic development, organ formation during fetal development, normal immune functions, and eye development and vision. The overconsumption of preformed vitamin A can be highly toxic and is especially contraindicated prior to and during pregnancy as it can result in severe birth defects. The tolerable upper intake level (UL) for vitamin A in adults is set at 3,000 mcg RAE/day. The UL does not apply to vitamin A derived from carotenoids. Vitamin A is a generic term that encompasses a number of related compounds (Figure 5). Retinol and retinyl esters are often referred to as preformed vitamin A. Retinol can be converted by the body to retinal, which can be in turn be oxidized to retinoic acid, the form of vitamin A known to regulate gene transcription. Retinol, retinal, retinoic acid, and related compounds are known as retinoids. β-Carotene and other food carotenoids that can be converted by the body into retinol are referred to as pro-vitamin A carotenoids. Hundreds of different carotenoids are synthesized by plants, but only about 10% of them are capable of being converted to retinol [3]. The following discussion will focus mainly on preformed vitamin A compounds and retinoic acid [21, 22].

CONCLUSION

If milk is missing from the diet then calcium intake can be increased with soy, rice milk, tofu or kale fermented soy products and certain soy products contain phytoestrogens, help to mimic the natural estrogen found in body, leading to reproductive health difficulties. Mg must be increased in the diet with beans, tofu and pea nuts. Antioxidant vitamin E helps to eliminate some PMS problems. Vitamin B_6 aids in the metabolism of proteins and red blood cells and has been cited in numerous studies to relieve depression. Vitamin C and zinc are essential as they support the health of a woman's eggs and reproductive system. Nutritional intake of the long-chain PUFA's Eicosapentaenoic acid (EPA) and DHA is inversely related to sperm concentration and motility which however certainly correlated with the ingestion of the short-chain omega-3 PUFA α-linolenic acid (ALA; 18:3w3). Food supplementation during the post-conception weeks with the anti-oxidant Astaxanthin, long-chain PUFA as a source of energy to the mitochondria, carnitines, and the co-enzyme ubiquinone Q10 may improve embryogenesis, cytokenesis, and perhaps implantation. Hormones are secreted by endocrine glands and hormones are essential to the proper functioning of the reproductive system. Therefore, the wellness of the endocrine gland is a precursor to mature reproductive functioning and health. Vitamin A is linked to growth and it is now recommended that all pregnant and breast feeding women take supplements of vitamin A (as beta-carotene) (no more than 10,000 IUs per day) as well as vitamins D and C. Menstruating women must consume iron or risk anemia; although this important mineral is widely taken in multivitamin form, your body will absorb iron better if you consume it in foods like spinach, lentils, lean red meat and dark poultry. If you are taking a multivitamin, make sure it is one made specifically for woman that includes iron. According to researchers, having sources of foods that are rich in selenium is something that gives visible outcomes for the male reproductive system. It activates selenoprotein that leads to good health of the sperm cells and enhance the reproductive system.

ACKNOWLEDGMENT

I am indebted to the morale support provided by my mother Smt. Rampyari Nautiyal, my brothers; Pradeep Nautiyal and Kishor Nautiyal, my sisters; Smt. Rekha S. Sharma, and Smt. Laxmi J. Manori. My wife Smt. Bhawna Nautiyal also deserves special thanks for her support.

REFERENCES

[1] *Women's Health* [Internet]. Available from: http://www.womens-health.co.uk/diet_repro_system.html.

[2] Martin GB, Rodger J, Blache D. Nutritional and environmental effects on reproduction in small ruminants. *Reprod Fertil Dev*.2004;16:491-501.

[3] Wade GN, Jones J. E. Neuroendocrinology of nutritional infertility. *Am JPhysiol Regul Integr Comp Physiol*.2014;287:R1277-R1296.

[4] Bronson FH. *Mammalian Reproductive Biology*. Chicago, IL: University of Chicago Press; 1989. 325pp.

[5] Comhaire FH, Decleer W. The Benefit of Nutraceutical Food Supplementation and Antioxidants for the Treatment of the Infertile Couple and in Assisted Reproduction. *Reproductive Sys Sexual Disord*. 2012; S1: 004. http://dx.doi.org/10.4172/2161-038X.S1-004.

[6] Comhaire F. The role of food supplementation in the treatment of the infertile couple and for associated reproduction. *Andrologia* 2010; 42:332-340.

[7] Nuble CJ. *Health guidance for better health* [Internet]. [Place unknown]. Available from: http://www.healthguidance.org/entry/35/1/Vitamins-and-Minerals-for-a-Healthy-Reproductive-System.html.

[8] *Ayurvedic Cure* [Internet]. Available from: http://www.ayurvediccure.com/5-best-diet-for-male-reproductive-system/.

[9] Beyene J, Han Z, Liao G, Mulla S, McDonald SD. Knowledge Synthesis Group. Maternal underweight and the risk of preterm birth and low birth weight: a systematic review and meta-analyses. *Int J Epidemiol*. 2011; 40(1): 65-101.

[10] Nohr EA, Vaeth M, Rasmussen S, Ramlau-Hansen CH, Olsen J. Waiting time to pregnancy according to maternal birth weight and pre pregnancy BMI. *Hum Reprod*. 2009; 24(1):226-232.

[11] Siega-Riz AM, King JC. Position of the American Dietetic Association and American Society for Nutrition: obesity, reproduction, and pregnancy outcomes. *J Am Diet Assoc*. 2009; 109(5):918-927.

[12] Clark AM, Ledger W, Galletly C, Tomlinson L, Blaney F, Wang X et al. Weight loss results in significant improvement in pregnancy and ovulation rates in ovulatory obese women. *Hum Reprod*. 1995; 10(10): 2705-2712.

[13] Chavarro JE, Toth TL, Wright DL, Meeker JD, Hauser R. Body mass index in relation to semen quality, sperm, DNA integrity, and serum reproductive hormone levels among men attending an infertility clinic. *Fertil Steril*. 2010; 93(7):2222-2231.

[14] NEDA. *Feeding Hope*, New York, [Internet]. Available from: www.national eatingdisorders.org.

[15] *ANRED* [Internet]. Available from: www.anred.com.

[16] Lucero J, Harlow BL, Barbieri RL, Sluss P, Cramer DW. Early follicular phase hormone levels in relation to patterns of alcohol, tobacco, and coffee use. *Fertil Steril*. 2001; 76:723-9.

[17] Ruiz-Luna AC, Salazar S, Aspajo NJ, Ribio J, Gasco M, Gonzales GF. Lepidium meyenii (Maca) increased litter size in normal adult female mice. *Reprod Biol Endocrinol*. 2005; 3: 16.

[18] Food and Nutrition Board, Institute of Medicine. *Vitamin A. Dietary Reference Intakes for Vitamin A, Vitamin K, Arsenic, Boron, Chromium, Copper, Iodine, Iron, Manganese, Molybdenum, Nickel, Silicon, Vanadium, and Zinc*. Washington, D.C.: National Academy Press; 2001. pp.65-126. [National Academy Press]

[19] Linus Pauling Institute. *Macronutrient Information Centre* [Internet]. Available from:http://lpi.oregonstate.edu/mic/vitamins/vitamin-A.

[20] WHO. *Guideline - Vitamin A supplementation in pregnant women*. Geneva: World Health Organization; 2011.

[21] Bozzo P, Chua-Gocheco A, Einarson A. Safety of skin care products during pregnancy. *Can Fam Phys*. 2011; 57(6):665-667.

[22] Gonzales GF, Cordova A, Gonzales C, Chung A, Vega K, Villena A. Lepidium meyenii (Maca) improved semen parameters in adult men. *Asian J Androl*.2001; 3: 301-303.

In: Diets and Diseases: Causes and Prevention
Editor: Wenbiao Wu

ISBN: 978-1-63484-580-9

Chapter 5

DIET AND LIVER DISEASES: A REVIEW OF CONTRIBUTING FACTORS

Huanhuan Zhang and Wenbiao Wu*
College of Food Science, Beibei, Chongqing, PRC

ABSTRACT

A safe diet is very important for preventing human body from liver injury. Many risk factors of liver injury could be present in human diets. They have been therefore analyzed.

It is concluded that our daily diets or foods contains several identified factors of damaging liver. These factors include over- or under-intake of some nutrients (including over-intake of energy, under-intake of protein/energy, over-intake of ethyl alcohol, over-intake of vitamin A, over-intake of niacin, over-intake of iron, over-intake of fluoride, and under- and over-intake of selenium), safrole, capsaicinoids, coumarin, gossypol, pyrrolizidine alkaloids, cycasin, heterocyclic amines, hydrazines, pyrones, pennyroyal oil, tannins, saponins, and contaminants.

Over-intake of energy and under-intake of protein/energy are especially significant because they are related to our staple foods or diets and therefore linked with daily diets or nutrition throughout life time. Heterocyclic amines are produced from meats during high temperature cooking. These risk factors are particularly significant for people who are used to eating meats as staple foods and cook meats by grilling, frying or baking. The risk factors including over-intake of vitamin A, over-intake of niacin, over-intake of iron, over-intake of fluoride, and under- and over-intake of selenium could also be very significant because they are linked with daily diets or nutrition throughout one's lifetime. Tannins and saponins may have beneficial and adverse effect on health depending on their dosage. Others may be considered as toxins.

So many risk factors of liver injury could exist in foods. The cooperative effects of the risk factors that are present in one's customary daily diet need to be studied well even though the concentration of each factor might be safe for consumption. Does any unknown risk factor of liver injury exist in foods?

* Corresponding Author Address: College of Food Science, Southwest University, 216 Tian Sheng Qiao, Beibei, Chongqing, PRC, Email: wbwu62@yahoo.com.

INTRODUCTION

Nowadays, the morbidity of liver diseases still appears to be a great contributor of global burden of morbidity and mortality [1]. For example, the same author also stated that only liver cirrhosis was estimated to cause 31.027 million Disability Adjusted Life Years (DALYs) (accounting for 1.2% of all DALYs, the DALYs accounting for all DALYs for males being 2 times that for females) and >1 million deaths (1.0308 million deaths accounting for 2.0% of all deaths, the deaths accounting for all deaths for males being 1.71 times that for females) in 2010 in the world. The DALY was defined as the addition of years of life lost to disability and to premature mortality by the author, which was used to estimate the burden of disease. Liver cancer caused additional 19.111 million DALYs (accounting for 0.8% of all DALYs, the DALYs accounting for all DALYs for males being 2 times that for females) and 0.7521 million deaths (accounting for 1.4% of all deaths, the deaths accounting for all deaths for males being 1.80 times that for females).

The illness of the human body may result from viral or bacterial infection, physical damage, genetic inheritance or mutation, intake of toxic compounds, over- or under-intake of essential nutrients or an unbalanced diet [2, 3]. The etiology of liver diseases should also be associated with the causes just mentioned above.

Among the causes, physical damage might occur rarely. Viral or bacterial infection looks as if it is not related to a diet. However, this may not be true. For example, it was reported that primary hepatocellular carcinoma was associated with interactions between the consumption of alcohol consumption and infections of hepatitis B and C infections [4]. Therefore, the evaluation of risk factors in human diets (including toxins and unbalanced nutrients in foods and over- or under-intake of some nutrients) is essential for the prevention or even the treatment of some chronic diseases [5].

Here, the risk factors of liver injury in human diets are summarized. This review could contribute greatly to the development of food science and technology as well as medicine, especially providing a theoretical basis of producing healthy food products, and guide individual's self-medication or nutritional management.

OVER- OR UNDER-INTAKE OF SOME NUTRIENTS

Over- or under-intake of some nutrients could increase the risk of liver diseases. Usually, these nutrients are taken daily. Therefore, the improper intake of these nutrients frequently occurs in the world.

Over-Intake of Energy

An excessive energy intake > 0 can cause overweight or obesity (Figure 1) and the mechanism that causes it was well discussed in the literature [6].

Obesity or being overweight can increase the risk of developing non-alcoholic fatty liver (or hepatic steatosis i.e., the amount of intracellular fat accounting for >5% of hepatocytes). This is due to the accumulation of fat in the liver [7]. This kind of liver disease commonly prevails in developed countries. For example, the morbidity of non-alcoholic fatty liver was found to be 27% to 38% of population in Western countries [8, 9] while that was 17% (15% in females and 19% in males) with about 90% of the patients requiring bariatric surgery in USA [10, 11]. Some individuals with non-alcoholic fatty liver (15 to 30%) can develop into advanced fibrosis, and 12 to 35% of which can further develop into cirrhosis [12] though it was not found to link with an elevated risk of all-cause mortality [13]. Furthermore, a non-alcoholic fatty liver was found to increase the risk of developing cardiovascular diseases [12]. It may not be necessary to believe that every case of fatty liver can cause a damage. But, sometimes the excessive accumulation of fat can result in the inflammation of the liver (or named steatohepatitis). A liver damage may result from this condition.

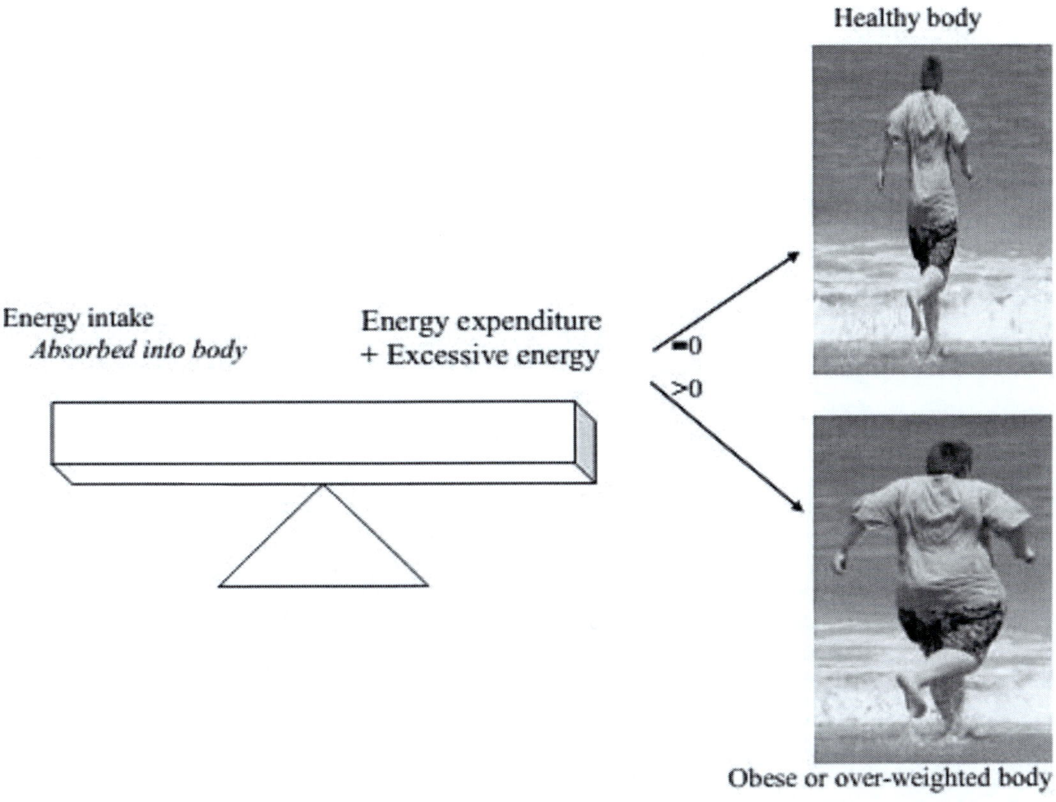

Figure 1. The key factor for energy balance and control of body weight.

The symptoms of nonalcoholic fatty liver disease may include pruritus, jaundice, and right upper quadrant pain [7]. The etiology of non-alcoholic fatty liver disease may involve in the induction of oxidative stress, the release of inflammatory cytokines, steatosis, and insulin resistance, leading to cirrhosis and fibrosis [14, 15], though further studies may be required to confirm its exact mechanism.

The energy-supplying compounds mainly include fats or oils (9 kcal/g), digestible saccharides (or named carbohydrates; 4 kcal/g), and alcohol (ethanol; 7 kcal/g). Proteins and amino acids (4 kcal/g) can also be oxidized as energy compounds if their supply is over the requirement of the body. Also, glycerol can be utilized to provide energy, which is a component of fats or oils.

Under-Intake of Protein/Energy

A damage and impaired function of the liver can result from an energy deficiency (or called under-intake of energy), no matter the cause. Figure 2 shows kwashiorkor which is caused by lack of protein and usually seen in underdeveloped countries. Fatty liver (the accumulation of fat in the liver) is one of symptoms observed in this disorder.

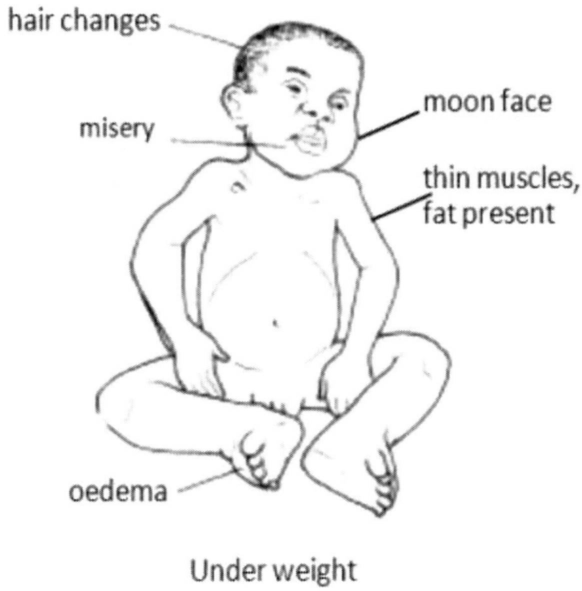

Figure 2 Kwashiorkor.

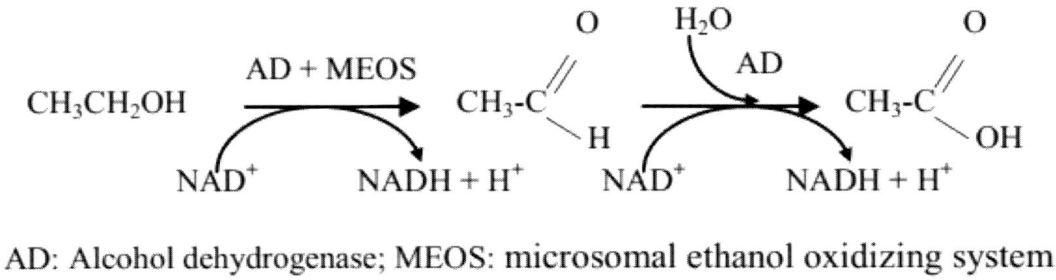

Figure 3. Metabolism of ethyl alcohol in the liver.

Diets with a lack of proteins or amino acids can cause this disease even though they supply enough energy. Furthermore, proteins or amino acids can be utilized as a source of energy and not play their primary functional role in maintenance or growth when the total intake of energy is too low. This can also result in kwashiorkor. A recent review paper indicated that severe malnutrition, including inadequate intake of protein, energy, and other nutrients can also result in liver injury in adults [16]. The author also stated that all stages of chronic liver disease are associated with the malnutrition of protein-calorie. It is essential to recognize the deficiency of macro or micronutrients as early as possible since the risk of complications can be reduced by the supplementation of nutrients.

Over-Intake of Ethyl Alcohol

It is consistently believed that the over-intake of ethyl alcohol (ethanol) increases the risk of developing all liver diseases [17]. It was reported that great portions of all liver diseases are contributed by alcoholic liver cirrhosis (ALC) and other alcoholic liver diseases (ALD) while >75% of all liver cirrhosis was found to be associated with the over-intake of ethyl alcohol in 2004 in the EU [18].

The mechanism of association of ethyl alcohol over-intake with the development of liver diseases may link to the production of acetaldehyde and the great demand of limited NAD^+ when it is metabolized (Figure 3). First, acetaldehyde is able to damage the liver. Second, a certain amount of ethyl alcohol in the cell heavily consumes NAD^+ (a coenzyme derived from niacin) whose supply is quite limited, and consequently reduces the NAD^+/NADH ratio. This can curtail other reactions dependent on NAD^+. For example, the speed of converting lactate to pyruvate by oxidation can be greatly slower, comparing with the reverse reaction. Then, the accumulation of lactate can be observed. Furthermore, other redox reactions dependent on NAD^+ can also similarly be slowed down in the tricarboxylic acid cycle. These can result in that <25% of the maximum rate of acetate oxidized, comparing with the normal condition. For this reason, the acetate is diverted into the system of synthesizing fatty acid. This can cause an alcoholic fatty liver. In a serious condition, liver cirrhosis and even cancer can be induced.

It should be noted that the adverse effect of ethyl alcohol intake on liver health in the human body is largely dependent on its dosage. An appropriate amount of ethyl alcohol intake may have beneficial effects on human health though large amount of intake is harmful. Therefore, drinking an appropriate amount of ethyl alcohol is generally accepted in the world. The critical question is that how much can be considered as being appropriate. Different countries may have different recommended maximum daily intake of alcoholic beverages, for example, 20 g (ethyl alcohol)/day in Australia, 20-24 g/day in Switzerland, 24 g/day in Czech Republic and Austria, 24-32 g/day in United Kingdom, 37 g/day in Portugal, 40 g/day in Italy, etc. [19]. OECD SIDS reported that about 2.4 g/kg bw/day in rats was the lowest reported the no observed adverse effect level (NOAEL) of ethyl alcohol intake and 3.600 g/kg bw/day or above caused adverse liver effects though it was stated that these data were not intended to be applied to alcoholic beverages [20].

Over-Intake of Vitamin A

The association of vitamin A intake with liver diseases has been reported in the literature though it is an essential nutrient for normal vision, reproduction and the immune system. For example, intake of vitamin A (retinol) at doses >100,000 IU (1IU = 0.3μg)/day was reported to cause liver injury [21]. Furthermore, a far lower dose (25,000 IU)/day of vitamin A was reported to cause severe hepatotoxicity [22].

The symptoms of toxicity should vary with the variation of excessive degree of vitamin A exposure and, therefore, extent of injury or damage in the liver. For example, few symptoms may be observed in the case of mild damage in the liver whereas liver failure may be caused ultimately by severe damage. The different severity of the excessive vitamin A exposure may cause the symptoms related to acute, subacute or chronic toxicities, respectively.

The etiology of the toxicity caused by over-intake of vitamin A is likely to initiate when it is stored in Ito cells. The Ito cells are believed to be "fat storing cells" whose cytoplasm frequently stores abundant amount of fats. The fatty substances include different varieties of lipids. Vitamin A is primarily stored in Ito cells. Vitamin A can induce the proliferation of this kind of cells. Toxic doses of vitamin A in the Ito cells (the facultative fibroblasts) can induce them to synthesize collagen which results in the fibrosis of the space of Disse. The exact mechanism of association of vitamin A over-intake with liver diseases may also involve in the excessive demand on microsomal enzymes which accelerate its metabolism (hyperprovitaminosis toxicity prevented and parts of pathological alterations in the liver reversed by increasing the activity of these enzymes), quick hemolysis of erythrocytes, and the alteration of lysosomes or mitochondria in the liver [23].

Generally, it is relatively uncommon to observe a liver damaged by vitamin A from our daily diet. This is due to the following reasons. Doses ≥1500 μg (5,000 IU)/day of vitamin A, which is far lower than that causing hepatotoxicity mentioned above in the first paragraph of this section, were reported to double the risk of hip fracture [24]. Especially, the Estimated Average Requirements (EAR), Recommended Dietary Allowances (RDA) (or Adequate Intake; AI) and Tolerable upper intake levels (UL) of vitamin A for adults were suggested to be 625, 900 and 3000 μg/day, respectively [25]. Therefore, a normal daily intake of vitamin A should not reach the amount that can cause hepatotoxicity. However, the long term intake of vitamin A supplements and foods very rich in carotenes (for example, yellow carote containing 3.62 mg/100 g fresh weight, spinach containing 3.87 mg/100 g fresh weight) should be cautious of its excessive supply.

The risk of inducing liver diseases and the severity of the symptoms in individuals may be modified by such factors as underlying liver problems, overall health, gender, race, ages, and genes.

Over-Intake of Niacin

Some scientific evidence appears to show that the over-intake of a certain amount of niacin is associated with liver damage. For example, it was reported that an i.p. dose of 500 mg/kg bw/day induced the glycogen deposition and enlargement of liver cells and the elevation of total hepatic lipids by about 50% and that a diet containing 0.5% nicotinamide or 2% nicotinic acids caused an increase of fatty acids by 4.3 – 15.8% or 4.2 - 11..8%, respectively in the liver of rats [26]. The authors also stated that it is generally believed that niacin doses >3 g/day for adults are potentially toxic. Furthermore, a dose of 9 g/day nicotinamide caused hepatic toxicity in a schizophrenic man [27].

On the other hand, a dose of about 300 mg/kg bw/day which was lower than the toxic doses mentioned in the above paragraph was found to ameliorate the hepatotocixity of carbon tetrachloride [28]. Long term experiments (12 months) on the doses of 200 mg/day to 3.5 g/day (equivalent to 50 mg/kg) did not show adverse effects [26].

The ERA, RDA and UL of niacin were suggested to be 12 mg/day (applied to men) (or 11 mg/day applied to women), 18 mg/day and 35 mg/day, respectively for adults [29]. For individuals with younger ages, the ERA, RDA and UL of niacin were lower, comparing with that for adults just mentioned above.

The amounts of some foods supplying niacin intake ≥35 mg/day are as the following: 228.78 g/day raw pork liver, 219.73 g/day Spanish peanuts, or 129.63 g/day defatted peanuts (calculated according to the data published by USDA [30]. The intake of this kind of foods should be cautious. Especially, foods rich in both niacin and tryptophan (convertible into niacin in the body) should be very cautious of evaluating toxicity. Furthermore, doses of 1000 – 2000 mg/day were suggested to treat cardiovascular diseases. These doses are much higher that the UL of niacin. It appears to be difficult to find a report on hepatic toxicity caused by these doses though ≥1000 mg/day niacin intake could cause other health problems [31].

Over-Intake of Iron

The function, and even structure of the liver, can be adversely affected by iron overload in the blood though other organ or tissues may be affected simultaneously. For example, it was reported that iron overload induced oxidative damage to lipids which linked to the dysfunctions of mitochondria and lysosomes and, therefore, hepatic mitochondrial respiration or calcium homeostasis may be adversely affected [32].

Iron storage in the human body is normally 200-1500 mg [33]. When Ferritin levels >1000 mcg/L in serum it may be considered as iron overload [34]. Another method of measuring iron overload is to measure iron content in liver. More than 7 mg Fe/g dry weight of liver is considered as iron overload [34].

Normally, dietary intake of iron is unlikely to result in iron overload in a health body since feedback mechanisms can restrict the absorption of iron by increases in storage iron [35]. However, iron overload may easily occur in individuals with primary hemochromatosis and ineffective erythropoiesis (HFE), which results from repetitive transfusions, hemoglobinopathies, and melodysplastic syndromes. The most common mutation gene (C282Y) is carried by about 10% of white population. HFE may occur in 4.4/1000 of these white people though it is not usually observed in other ethnic people [36]. During the treatment of HFE, a diet containing certain amount of vitamin C and irons is harmful [6].

The ERA, RDA and UL of iron were suggested to be 6 mg/day (applied to men) (or 8.1 mg/day applied to women), 8 mg/day (applied to men) (or 18 mg/day, applied to women) and 45 mg/day, respectively, for adults [25].

The amounts of some foods supplying iron intake ≥45 mg/day are as the following: 101.11 g/day raw beef spleen, 107.41 g/day raw lamb spleen, 201.61 g/day raw pork spleen, or raw pork liver (calculated according to the data published by USDA [30]. An intake of canned drinks or foods in a poorly tined can should also be cautious of causing iron toxicity. An intake of >50 mg/day iron may cause serious acute toxicity. Acute toxicity of iron may undergo 5 stages: 1, gastrointestinal distress, 2, latent period, 3, metabolic/cardiovascular symptoms, 4, hepatic dysfunction or damage, and 5, delayed period. Intake of iron supplements should be very cautious of causing serious acute toxicity.

Over-Intake of Fluoride

Scientific evidences indicate that over-intake of fluoride is able to cause hepatic toxicity. For example, an experimental study concluded that drinking water containing 500 mg/L sodium fluoride (226 mg/L fluoride ion) caused increases in the activities of serum transaminase (alanine transaminase; aspartate transaminase) (biomarkers of liver dysfunction or damage), high levels of malondialdehyde in the liver (markers of lipid oxidation), and the infiltration of mononuclear cells, hepatocellular necrosis or extensive ballooning in the liver, comparing with controls [37]. Furthermore, another study concluded that 10 mg/L/kg bw sodium fluoride by oral administration caused few focal areas in liver, necrosis of hepatic cells, proliferation of hepatic cords, distorted hepatic cords with necrosis, vacuolated hepatic cells, enlarged and dilated hepatic vein with degeneration of hepatocyte and excessive hepatic cell necrosis [38]. Intake of fluoride at high doses was found to adversely alter the metabolism, function, and structure of liver and kidney [39].

The AI and UL of fluoride were suggested to be 4 mg/day (applied to men) (or 3 mg/day applied to women) and 10 mg/day, respectively, for adults [40] whereas 7 mg/day was recommended to be its UL for adults by EFSA [41].

It is normally rare to result in excessive intake of fluoride through diets alone since most common foods contain only a small amount of it. However, multiple sources of exposure could cause accumulative fluoride toxicity. Drinking large amounts of water (especially that rich in fluoride) in combination with the intake of foods grown in some coal-producing areas or with fluoride-laden fertilisers, or low protein diets and the over-use of tooth paste may greatly elevate the intake of fluoride.

Under- and Over-Intake of Selenium

It was reported that selenium deficiency was associated with cirrhosis [42]. Another study also tended to indicate the association of selenium deficiency with liver diseases [43, 44]. The mechanism of association of selenium deficiency with liver diseases may link to elevated lipoperoxidation and reduced glutathione levels in the liver. On the other hand, a patient developed congestion of the kidneys and liver, hemorrhagic stomach mucosa, and pulmonary edema, after taking approximately 90 mL of gun-bluing with 4% selenious acid (liver selenium found to be 5.4 μg/g wet wt) [45].

The ERA, RDA and UL of selenium were suggested to be 45 μg/day, 55 μg/day and 400 μg/day, respectively, for adults [46]. It should be noted that, the ERA and RDA are different for children, people with old ages, pregnant or lactating women.

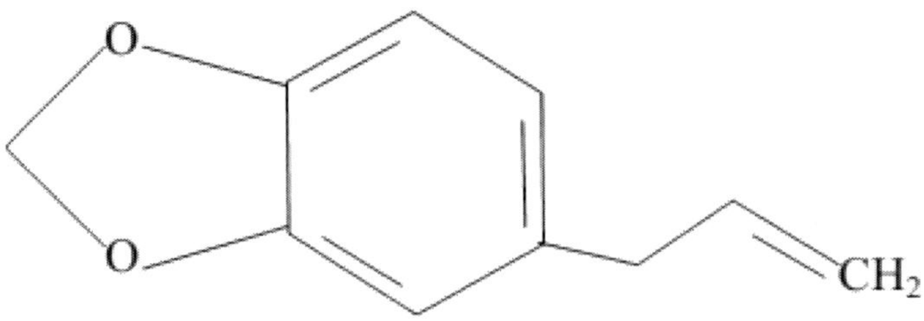

Figure 4. Diagram of molecular structure of safrole.

In only limited areas, for example, the high-selenium areas of Wyoming and South Dakota in USA, Enshi of Hubei or Ziyang of Shanxi in China, there is a risk of ingesting selenium over the UL. On the other hand, in vast areas for example, most places in China, there is a risk of selenium deficiency.

SAFROLE

Scientific evidences consistently show that safrole is able to cause hepatic damage. For example, doses at 250 – 750 mg/kg bw/day were found to cause liver alterations: the proliferation of bile duct, the enlargement of cells, fatty metamorphosis, cystic necrosis, and adenomatoid hyperplasia [47]. Long term toxicity studies indicated that safrole had the properties of inducing liver cancer [48, 49].

Therefore, safrole and sassafras were banned by the US Food and Drug Administration (FDA) though in that time safrole was still considered as a weak carcinogen compound by FDA [50]. SCF concluded that safrole has been found to be carcinogenic and genotoxic, that it is not able to assume the existence of a threshold and a safe exposure limit could not be established, and that consequently, the exposure should be reduced and the use levels should be restricted [51]. It appears that the UL of safrole has not been established.

Safrole, a phenylpropene has typically been found in the seeds of black pepper (Piper Nigrum L.). It is also present in other varieties of herbs and spices, for example, nutmeg, cinnamon, mace, and basil. It is very rich in long pepper [52]. The diagram of its structure is shown in Figure 5.

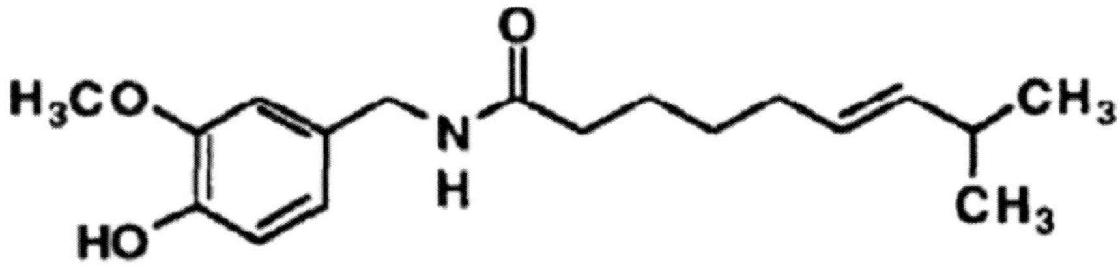

Figure 5. Diagram of molecular structure of capsaicin.

CAPSAICINOIDS

Some evidence appears to indicate the hepatic toxicity of capsainoids though more researches may be required for establishing the complete information about their toxicity. For example, it was found that 50 μg capsaicin (one of capsainoids) with alcoholic chilli extract (20 μl) (equivalent to about 0.5 mg/kg bw/day) increased histopathological lesions in liver (mainly liver cirrhosis) and other organs as well as mortality, comparing with controls (20 μl alcohol) [53]. Furthermore, 10% chillies added to a semisynthetic diet with the presence of ardein (a purified ground nut protein) caused neoplastic alterations in the liver (hepatomas, adenocarcinomas or solid adenomas of the bile duct, multiple cystic cholangiomas) [54]. SCF tends to conclude that capsaicin is potentially carcinogenic though controversial argument exists [55]. It also appears that, in addition of damaging liver, capsainoids are simultaneously toxic to other organs or tissues when over-ingested [56-60].

It seems that there is limited information about the mechanism of toxicity of capsaicinoids. However, the interaction of capsaicin with xenobiotic metabolizing enzymes (especially monooxygenases dependent on microsomal cytochrome P450) may be associated with the activation of some mutagens and carcinogens. Hepatic cytochrome P450 2El is involved in the catalysis of converting capsaicin to reactive species for example the phenoxy radical intermediate. This kind of intermediate is able to covalently bind to the active site of the enzyme and tissue macromolecules. The alteration of nucleic acids and protein by the covalent binding can result in carcinogenesis, mutagenesis, and necrosis.

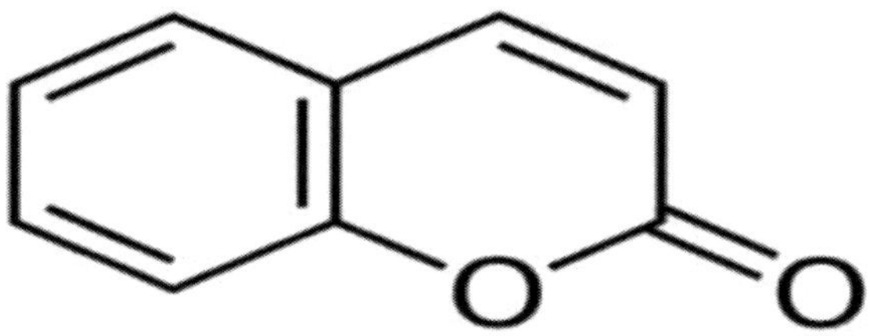

Figure 6. Diagram of molecular structure of coumarin.

Since capsaicin is frequently used as a medicine and food additive, complete safety evaluation of this compound would be necessary [61]. The LD_{50} of capsaicin in male mice ranges 0.56 mg/kg bw (i.v.) to 60 – 75 mg/kg bw (in ethanol) or 190 (122 – 294) mg/kg bw (in dimethyl sulfoxide) [55]. However, it appears that the UL or NOAEL of this compound or other capsaicinoids has not been established yet.

Capsaicin (8-methyl-N-vanillyl-6-nonenamide; its structural diagram shown in Figure 5) is the principle irritating and pungent component in red peppers and chilies which are frequently consumed as spices or even vegetables in many parts of the world, for example, southwest China. Oleoresin red pepper and chilli pepper typically contain 60 mg/g and 0.1 - 2.5 mg/g capsaicinoids, respectively [62]. It was also reported that 0.22 - 20 mg total capsaicinoids/g by dry weight were present in varieties of peppers, for example, Capsicum frutescens, annuumand chinensewere [63]. Dihydrocapsaicin and capsaicin were found to be 0.83 and 1.32 mg/g by dry weight in cayenne pepper samples, respectively [64]. Therefore, the consumption of these foods should be very cautious of causing toxicity.

COUMARIN

It is almost consistently reported that coumarin is able to damage liver. The lowest dose of coumarin capable of causing hepatic damage was reported to be 0.4 mg/kg bw/day [65], which may however be reversible [66]. Furthermore, intake of certain amount of coumarin may cause hepatic and pulmonary toxicity that can induce liver and lung tumours [67]. Many other reports on the hepatic toxicity of coumarin can be found in the literature [68-72].

The mechanism of association of ingesting coumarin with hepatic damage may link to its conversion to its metabolites (for example, coumarin 3,4-epoxide intermediate) which is toxic [73]. The conversion of coumarin to its metabolites needs cytochrome P450-dependent enzymes. This conclusion is supported by the fact that cytochrome P450 inhibitors (for example, metyrapone and ellipticine) can inhibit the toxicity of coumarin. It seems that glutathione (GSH) covalently react with the toxic coumarin metabolite(s) to form conjugates and therefore ameliorate the toxicity. This may be the reason that depleted nonprotein sulfhydryl groups (mainly decrease in glutathione (GSH)) in liver is usually observed when toxicity is induced by coumarin. This alteration should not be the outcome of forming oxidized glutathione (GSSG) or leaking out hepatocellular GSSG and/or GSH. The depletion of hepatocellular GSH by diethyl maleate can potentiate the toxicity of coumarin.

Based on experiments with dogs, it was estimated that 10 mg coumarin/kg bw)/day was the overall NOAEL for its toxicity in liver in the most species of sensitive animals. Therefore, EFSA (2008) recommended a Tolerable Daily Intake of 0 - 0.1 mg coumarin/kg bw by applying a safety factor of 100 [67].

Coumarin (see Figure 6) is found in cinnamon and many other plants. Ceylon (Cinnamomum zeylandicum) and Cassia cinnamon (Cinnamomum aromaticum) are the two main types of plants that contain significant amount of coumarin. Ceylon cinnamon is less frequently employed in preparing food products, comparing with Cassia cinnamon. This compound can also be present in apricots, woodruff, bison grass, cherries, strawberries, sweet clover, and tonka beans. Cassia cinnamon contains 90 - 12200 mg/kg coumarin while Ceylon cinnamon contains un-detectable level - 190 mg/kg [74, 75]. Another report also reported relative low level (<15 mg/kg) of coumarin in Ceylon cinnamon [75]. Too much supplementation of Cassia cinnamon in food products would very likely cause a health problem.

GOSSYPOL

It is consistently reported that gossypol can damage the liver [76-82]. Gossypol at dose of 25 mg/kg BW by a single intraperitoneal caused hepatocyte degeneration (strong nuclear pyknosis and cytoplasmic eosinophilia) in rats [78] while 30 mg/kg bw resulted in the same health problem [79]. Gossypol at doses of 30 mg/kg bw/day for two weeks or 15 mg/kg bw/day for four weeks resulted in morphological alterations of the liver in rats: proliferation of collagen fiber in the perisinusoidal space, an expanded perinuclear space, an enlarged endoplasmatic reticulum, and mitochondrial vacuolation, and observed by electron microscopy [81]. A diet containing 0.1% free gossypol elevated lipidosis and activity of gamma glutamyltransferase in plasma in the liver of chickens when fed for 21 days [77]. Furthermore, a diet containing 0.4% gossypol significantly decreased the liver weight of broilers when fed for 20 days [76]. Simultaneously, gossypol can damage other organs or tissues [83].

The mechanism of the hepatic toxicity of gossypol appears to need more researches to be established. However, biochemical analysis indicated that gossypol resulted in changes in the activity of seric enzymes, reduction of GSH levels and elevation of GSSG [84].

EFSA concluded that 0.1 mg/kg bw/day gossypol was the lowest dose currently identified to cause a health problem in human body and no ADI or TDI has yet been established [85]. Furthermore, the lowest dose of gossypol toxic to the liver has also not been identified. Further research related to this aspect would be worthwhile.

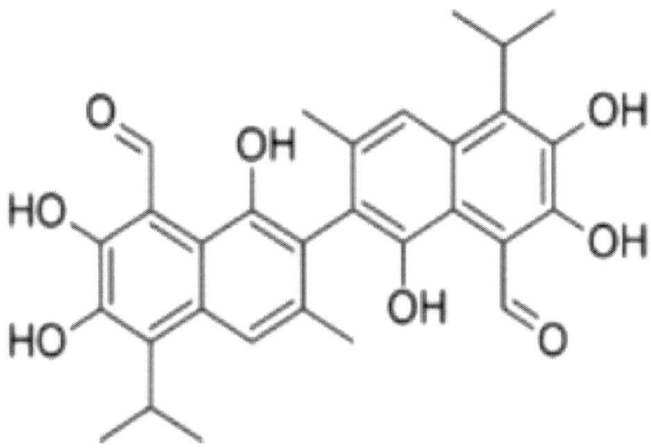

Figure 7. Diagram of molecular structure of gossypol.

Gossypol (Figure 7) is mainly found in cottonseeds. For example, 266,000 mg/kg (26.6%) total gossypol and 1,750 mg/kg (0.175%) free gossypol which is toxic are present in cottonseed meal (85). However, gossypol content may significantly vary with the variation of varieties. For example, its content in the seed of G. barbadense was reported to be up to 34 g/kg [86]. The proportions of (−) gossypol are 33.8 - 47.0% in the seeds of G. hirsutum [87, 88] and 24.9 - 68.9% in that of G. barbadense [86]. Therefore, the addition of cottonseed meal to food product should be very cautious of its toxicity. Also, unrefined cottonseed oil is likely to be toxic.

Pyrrolizidine Alkaloids

It is consistently reported that the liver was one of the main organs adversely targeted by pyrrolizidine alkaloids (PA; Figure 8). The toxicity of these compounds usually cause lesions in the liver (mostly confluent haemorrhagic necrosis, followed by in the central and sublobular veins (occlusion of the lumen, thrombosis, deposits of fibrin, necrosis, and subintimal oedema) [89]. A mixture of pyrrolizidine alkaloids (92% riddelliine, 5% retrorsine, 1.3% seneciphylline) at doses of 1.0 mg/kg and above elevated the morbidity of liver lesions (cytologic alterations, hepatocytic karyomegaly, and haemorrhagic centrilobular hepatic necrosis) and damage of other organs in male rats [90, 91]. ESFA concluded that the lowest identified doses for short-term intake able to cause hepatic veno-occlusive disease (HVOD) in humans are 3 mg PA/kg bw/day (for a boy) and 0.8 -1.7 mg PA/kg bw/day (for a girl), and that the lowest identified dose for long-term intake able to result in HVOD is 15 μg PA/kg bw/day [89]. PA toxicity can be reversible and complete recovery is possible if the liver damage is not too severe and its intake is stopped.

The exact mechanism of PA toxicity may need more researches to illustrate. However, PA intake was found to increase Cu, decrease Zn, cause abnormal metabolism of Fe with greatly impaired hematopoiesis in the liver, and alter metabolism of vitamin A (decreasing levels of vitamin A in the liver and plasma) [92]. Furthermore, for causing liver cancer, the primary site for genotoxicity caused by 1,2-unsaturated PA is in the liver. The 1,2-unsaturated PA from classes with different structures (mono-esters and di-esters; otonecine, heliotridine, and retronecine) is metabolized to pyrrolic intermediates which arereactive and a common set of DHP adducts is formed at dG and dA sites of DNA in rat liver, which propose a genotoxic carcinogenic mechanism applied to all 1,2-unsaturated-PA esters and their N-oxides that can be metabolically converted into PA [89].

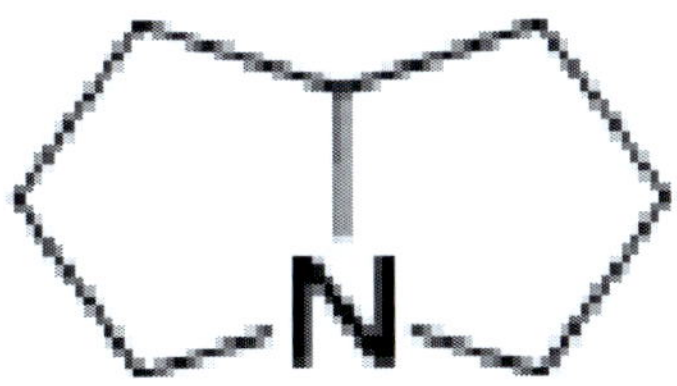

Figure 8. Diagram of basic molecular structure of PA. Many PAs are derived from this basic structure.

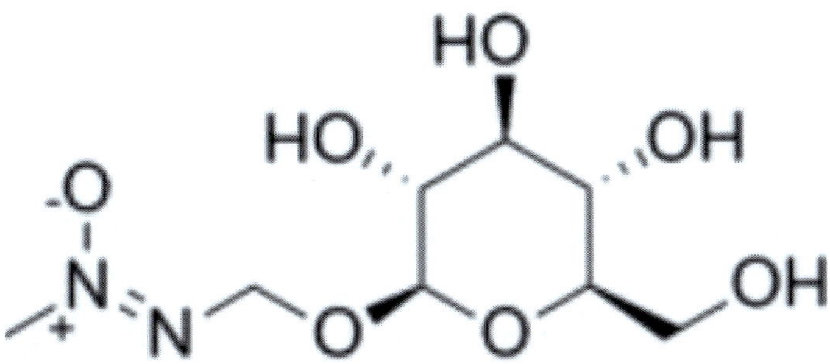

Figure 9. Diagram of molecular structure of cycasin.

It seems that the NOAEL, UL or TDI of PA have not been established. For safe consumption and evaluation of exposure risk, it would be worth carrying out further studies on this aspect.

Many foods or their products can be contaminated by PA. Among foods, PAs are mostly present in honey (concentrations of 0.5-1087 μg/kg reported) [89]. In plants, the seeds of contaminated forage or cereal crops sometimes contain PA. Flour and other foods may also be occasionally contaminated by PA. Milk can be contaminated if cows are fed with PA contaminated plants. Over 100 hepatotoxic PAs were isolated from *Leguminosae, Compositae*, and *Boraginaceae* families. Pollen samples from such plants as Echium spp., Eupatorium spp. and Senecio spp. were found to contain11-37,855 μg/kg PA [93]. PAs were also found in some herbal products, such as comfrey (genus Symphytum), borage (Family Boraginaceae), and 'gordolobo yerba' (Family Asteraceae) [94]. It was also reported that more than 350 PAs are identified, which exist in 6000 plant species (for example, Fabaceae(genus Crotalaria), Asteraceae (tribes Senecionae and Eupatoriae), and the families Boraginaceae(all genera), with concentrations of <0.001% - 5% in seeds of certain plant [89].

The hepatoxic PAs can adversely affect health in all humans. Large quantity intake of herbal teas and home remedies can increase the risk of PA poisonings. The only way to prevent PA toxicity is to avoid any products containing it.

CYCASIN

Cycasin at doses of 50–75 mg/kg bw/day was found to cause hepatocellular carcinoma when orally given for 5 days/week [95]. This compound is therefore hepatoxic and carcinogenic. The lowest dose of causing liver and other organ tumors in rats was published to be 2.5 mg cycasin/kg bw given by subcutaneous [96].

It seems that the NOAEL, UL andTDI of cycasin have not been established. For safe consumption and evaluation of exposure risk, it would be worth carrying out further studies on this aspect though its occurrence in foods or food products may be very limited.

Cycasin (Figure 9) mainly has been found in cycads for example Zamia pumila and Cycas revolute. The seeds of these plants usually have the highest concentration of cycasin though other parts can also contain it. It was also found that the larvae of insects fed on Z. pumila can also contain this toxin. Nowadays, cycads are not commonly planted as food crops. Therefore, the significance of exposure to this toxin through diet may be rare. However, if there is the application of cycads to the production of food or feed resources, its safety for consumption should be well evaluated.

HETEROCYCLIC AMINES

It is generally believed that heterocyclic amines (HCAs) are able to cause liver cancers. For example, it was reported that 2-amino-3,8-dimethylimidazo[4,5-f]quinoxaline (MeIQx), one of HCAs, at a total dose of 1.25 μmol (~266 μg) or 0.625 μmol (~133 μg)by i.p. injection induced liver tumors in male B6C3F1/nctr mice [97]. Several others also reported that other HCAs (for example, 2-amino-3,4-dimethylimidazo[4,5-f] quinoline(MeIQ), 2-Amino-1-methyl-6-phenylimidazo[4,5-b] pyridine (PhIP)) can cause liver diseases including tumors [98-102].

It seems that the NOAEL, UL andTDI of HCAs have not been established. For safe consumption and evaluation of exposure risk, it would be worth carrying out further studies on this aspect since its occurrence in cooked meats could be significant.

HCAs are usually produced during the preparation of muscle meats (for example, poultry, fish, pork, beef) by a method employing high temperature (for example, grilling over an open flame, pan frying), especially above 300°F [103]. For example, the concentration of part of HCAs (including PhIP, AαC, IQ, DiMeIQx and MeIQx) in beef steak cooked by broiling or frying at 150-225°C was found to be as high as 144.09 μg/kg [104]. The formation of HCAs involves the interaction of creatine (a substance found in muscle), sugars, and amino acids (the building blocks of proteins). The efficiency of forming HCAs during cooking may vary with the variation of varieties of meats. Barbecued, grilled, or over cooked steak and chicken may contain high levels of HCAs [105]. The types of HCAs isolated from cooked or heated fish or meat and structurally identified are more than ten though most of them are not previously registered compounds.

It is, therefore, recommended that exposure to HCAs should beavoided and that their biological effects should be reduced as far as possible. Supplementation of functional compounds, for example soy-isoflavones in foods and cooking by using microwave ovens may be able to inhibit the formation of HCAs. A proper guideline of about how to reduce the formation of HCAs during cooking or processing to the general public would be a vital way greatly contributing to the prevention of cancer [106].

HYDRAZINES

It is consistently believed that hydrazine can cause liver diseases. Although it appears to be difficult of finding toxicological studies on hydrazine by oral administration in the literature, there are several reports on its hepatic toxicity observed inhalation investigation. For example, continuous inhalation of 0.2 ppm hydrazine for 6 months was found to cause liver lesions in mice, monkeys, and dogs [107]. Liver damage (for example, necrosis and degeneration of the liver) by inhalation of hydrazine was also observed by others [108-110].

The mechanism of association of hydrazines with hepatic damage needs more researches to confirm. However, the metabolism of hydrazines to toxic intermediates by P450 may be associated with the mechanism of hydrazine toxicity to liver.

It seems that the NOAEL, UL andTDI of hydrazines have not been established. For safe consumption and evaluation of exposure risk, it would be worth carrying out further studies on this aspect since its occurrence in edible mushrooms could be significant.

Hydrazines (Figure 10) are mainly found in mushrooms (for example Gyromitra esculenta, and Agaricus bisporus) which are eaten commonly. For example, the concentration of β-N-(γ-L(+)-Glutamyl)-4-(hydroxymethyl) phenylhydrazine (agaritine) in Agaricus mushroom was found to be 112 - 1836 μg/g dry weight [111]. In addition to agaritine (a hydrazine derivative of an amino acid), several other derivatives (for example, gyromitrin) of hydrazine were also isolated from the most popular edible mushroom Agaricus bisporus [112]. The false morel, Gyromitra esculenta contains significant amount of hydrazines. For example, concentrations of 40 to 150 mg/kg monomethylhydrazine were found in the false morel [113]. Because hydrazines are quite volatile, their concentration in well cooked mushroom (especially dried mushroom) should be very limited. So well cooking is an efficient way to eliminate the toxicity caused by hydrazines in mushrooms. Person who continuously cooking mushrooms for a long term should be cautious of toxicity caused by the vapor of hydrazines.

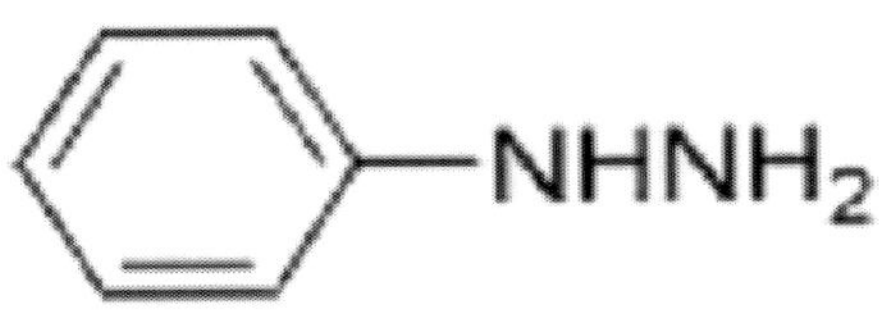

Figure 10. Diagram of basic molecular structure of hydrazine Many hydrazines are derived from this basic structure.

PYRONES

It is mostly believed that the pyrones in kava products can damage liver though controversial opinion also exists [114]. The liver toxicity of products supplemented with kava pyrones was reported by health-care professionals from the United States, Switzerland, and

Germany since 1999. For example, it was reported that the intake of products supplemented with kava pyrones caused severe damage to liver and that liver transplantation subsequently had to be implemented because of liver failure [115-121]. The Food and Drug Administration (FDA) published a guideline for consumers in response to the reports on five toxicity cases occurred (one in USA and four in Europe) [122]. FDA's report showed the investigation into the liver failure linked with the consumption of the products supplemented with kava pyrones in USA and the summary of the cases in Europe. Subsequently, an experimental study was completed, which showed an adverse effect of kava pyrones similar to the case previously reported in USA. Furthermore, it was reported that low doses of kava pyrones were able to cause liver toxicity which is dose dependent [123].

It seems that the NOAEL, UL andTDI of kava pyrones are currently absent from the literature. For safe consumption and evaluation of exposure risk, it would be worth carrying out further studies on this aspect since information about its occurrence in natural foods is very limited.

Kava pyrone products are isolated from the roots and rhizome of *Piper methysticum* (a shrub indigenous to the South Pacific). Kava pyrones-containing products are produced for being used as dietary supplement and for treating stress premenstrual syndrome, occasional insomnia, and anxiety. Concentrated extracts or raw plant materials are usually used as supplements. The diagram of basic molecular structure of Kava pyrones is shown in Figure 11. Many pyrone derivatives naturally exist. For example, 15 kava pyrones were identified. Some of them are generally substituted 5, 6-dihydro-alpha-pyrones or substituted alpha pyrones [124]. The basic unit of kava pyrone may also be named 4-methoxy-2-pyrones with phenyl or styryl substitutes [125].

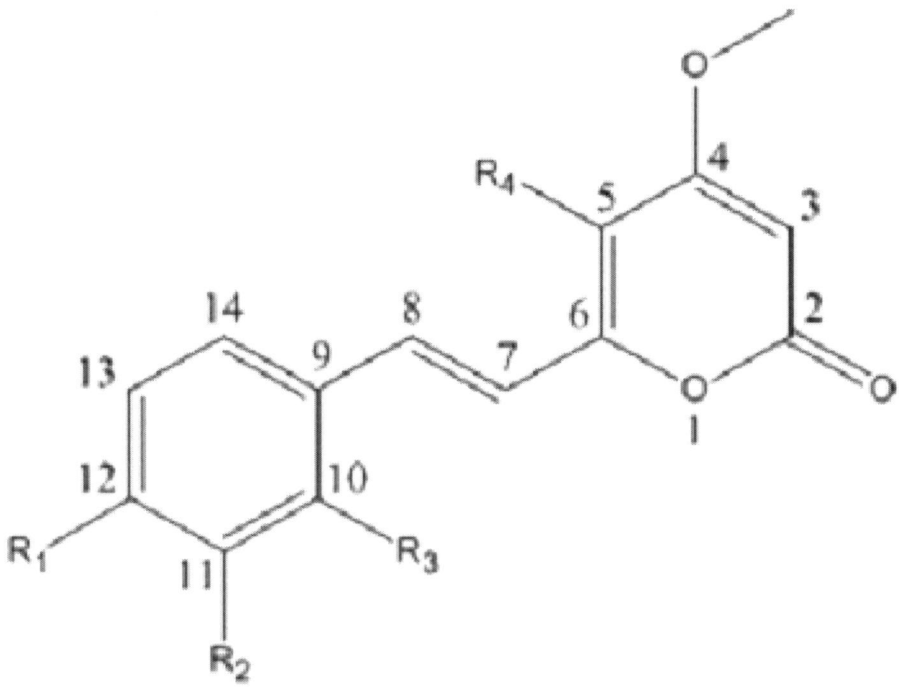

Figure 11. Diagram of basic molecular structure of pyrone. Many pyrones are derived from this basic structure.

Pennyroyal Oil

It is consistently believed that pennyroyal oil (Mentha pulegium) can cause liver damage. For example, it was reported that 10 ml pennyroyal oil (containing 62-97% pulegone, i.e., ca 5.4-9 g pulegone, ca 90-150 mg/kg bw for a 60 kg person calculated by using 0.9 as the relative density of peppermint oil) caused moderate to severe damage in the liver (massive centrilobular necrosis observed) and other health problems while >15 ml (containing ca 8-13 g pulegone, ca 130-215 mg/kg bw for a 60 kg person) caused death [126]. Chronic animal studies showed that liver and kidney were target organs for the toxicity of menthofuran and pulegone (the main component of pennyroyal oil) [127]. Pennyroyal oil that has 85% of pulegone is able to acutely result in multiorgan injury (for example liver necrosis) in studying animals.

The formation of reactive metabolites may be involved in the mechanism of toxicity of pulegone and menthofuran. This is also supported by recent *in vitro* experimental data obtained recently. For example, pulegone, the principal component in pennyroyal oil seems to be converted to intermediates that are toxic to the liver through the action of cytochrome P450 system (CYP 1A2 and 2E1). Depletion of glutathionine levels can be caused by pulegone and its products. The ability of N-acetyl cysteine and glutathionine to ameliorate the toxicity of pennyroyal may support this hypothesis.

The no effect level and TDI of pulegone were suggested to be 20 mg/kg bw/day and 0.1 mg/kg bw/day, respectively [128]. The no effect level and TDI of menthofuran are similar to that of pulegone.

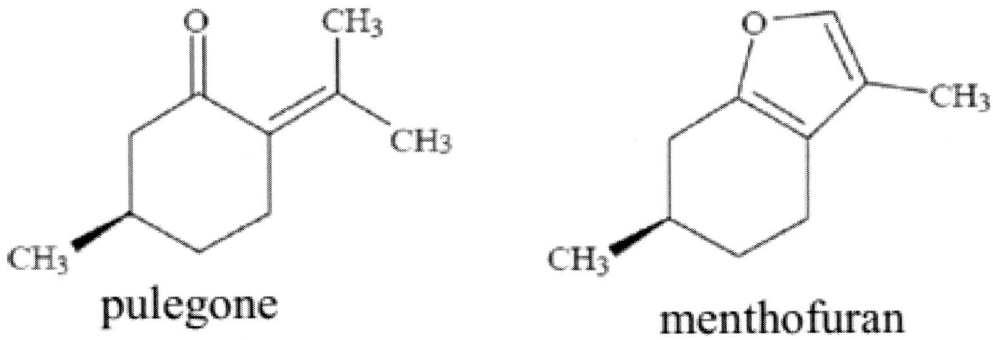

Figure 12. Diagram of molecular structure of pulegone and menthofuran.

It appears that reports on the cases of liver damaged by this oil still exist. It would be worth carrying out further studies on the evaluation of dietary safety, exposure doses and occurrence in foods or diets.

Tannins

It is generally believed that tannins are associated with the health of the liver. For example, it was reported that rhubarb tannins at higher doses of 14.69 g/kg bw and 40.00 g/kg bw aggravated liver fibrosis caused by CCl_4 though they at lower doses of 2.00 g/kg bw and

5.40 g/kg bw ameliorated liver damage (i.e., decreased the fibrosis)) caused by CCl_4 [129]. Furthermore, hydrolysable tannins abundantly found in vegetables (e.g., spinach), fruits (e.g., banana, persimmon), and beverages (e.g., red wine, tea, cocoa, coffee) were reported to be hepatotoxic in animals though their hepatic toxicity in human were rarely reported in the literature [130].

Contradistinctively, the hepatoprotective effects of tannins were also reported in the literature [131]. In this study, the samples tested are crude extracts or isolates. Maybe, it's worthwhile carrying out experimental studies on purified tannins.

The hepatotoxicity of tannins may vary with the variation of their origins or their molecular characteristics. Second, their doses used for the test or ingested may be critical for their hepatotoxicity. Apart to the hepatic properties of tannins per se, depleting the nutritional quality of some nutrients by the intake of large quantity of tannins might also be a concern. For example, tannins are able to decrease the digestibility of proteins or energy compounds and therefore can cause the deficiency of proteins (or essential amino acids)/energy in the body. This could cause liver diseases (*see Under-Intake of Protein/Energy*). Perhaps, the separation of nutrients and tannins and taking them separately are good attempts to take the advantages of functional properties of both. By this way, it would be easy to accurately control the dietary dosage of tannins and the interaction between them and digestive enzymes.

Saponins

Crude saponins from *Madhuca* were found to be hepatotoxic [132]. The LD_{50} of crude *Madhuca* saponins is 1.0 g/kg bw and at high doses they were found to be toxic to the liver, gastro-intestinal, and kidney. Pentacyclic triterpenoids are the main components of crude *Madhuca* saponins. Pentacyclic triterpenoids isolated from Lantana camara were also found to cause hepatotoxicity [133].

Conversely, there are also reports on the hepatoprotective effect of saponins [134]. So, what is the truth?

Perhaps, dosage is the critical factor for the toxicity of saponins. Second, impurity in the materials tested may also affect the outcome of studies.

It was reported that triterpenoids saponins at doses of 300 -750 mg/kg bw did not show adverse effects [135, 136]. It was also reported that steroidal saponins at an oral dose of 510 - 562.5 mg/kg bw were not found to be toxic [137]. The NOAEL, UL or TDI of saponins appears to be not established.

Saponins are found to be widely present in many food materials such as soybean, potato, quinoa, onion, and garlic. It seems that no report on the hepatotoxicity of saponins from these foods can be found in the literature. The content of saponins varies very much in different plants and even different organs within a plant. For example, it was found that the total concentration of saponin was 1.5-23 g/kg in seed crops for example soybean and quinoa, 100 g/kg in the seeds of Madhuca, 100-300 g/kg in licorice root or quillaja bark (138. The content of saponins was found to be about 5 g/kg in whole soybean seeds [139] or 5.1−7.0 g/kg in defatted soybean meal [140]. For safe consumption and evaluation of exposure risk, it would be worth carrying out further studies on the establishment of NOAEL, UL or TDI of saponins. This is also very important for the use of saponin rich materials as food resources and the proper utilization of saponins.

CONTAMINANTS

Contaminants, for example, heavy metals like mercury, lead, aluminium and arsenic or some micro-organisms from the environment could also elevate the risk of hepatic damage. If growing soil contains significant amount of the heavy metals, foods produced in the soil would also be significantly contaminated by them. Aflatoxins are usually released by micro-organisms: for example, *A. parasiticus* and *A. flavus*. There are also other hepatic toxins released by micro-organisms: for example, rubratoxin from *P. purpurogenum* and *P. rubrum,* phomopsin from *P. leptostromiformis,* and fumonisins from *F. proliferatum*, *F. moniliform* and *F. verticillioides*. Furthermore, some chemicals, for example, butylated hydroxytoluene, which are commonly used as food additives can also have hepatotoxicity.

CONCLUSION

It is concluded that our daily diets or foods contain several identified factors of damaging liver. These factors include over- or under-intake of some nutrients (including over-intake of energy, under-intake of protein/energy, over-intake of ethyl alcohol, over-intake of vitamin A, over-intake of niacin, over-intake of iron, over-intake of fluoride, and under- and over-intake of selenium), safrole, capsaicinoids, coumarin, gossypol, pyrrolizidine alkaloids, cycasin, heterocyclic amines, hydrazines, pyrones, pennyroyal oil, tannins, saponins, and contaminants.

Especially, over-intake of energy and under-intake of protein/energy are very significant because they are related to our staple foods or diets and therefore linked with daily diets or nutrition throughout life time. Heterocyclic amines are produced from meats during high temperature cooking. These risk factors are particularly significant for people who are used to eat meats as staple foods and cook meats by grilling, frying or baking. The risk factors including over-intake of vitamin A, over-intake of niacin, over-intake of iron, over-intake of fluoride, and under- and over-intake of selenium could also be very significant because they are linked with daily diets or nutrition throughout life time. Tannins and saponins may have beneficial and adverse effects on health depending on their dosage. Others may be considered as toxins.

For some risk factors of liver diseases, for example, UL has not yet been established. Therefore, it would be worth carrying out further studies on this aspect in future.

So many risk factors of liver injury could exist in foods. Their cooperative effects of the risk factors that are present in one's customary daily diets need to be studied well even though the concentration of each factor might be safe for consumption. Does any unknown risk factor of liver injury exist in foods? This should also be perspective research areas in future.

It is believed that this review is useful for the prevention of liver diseases in individuals by proper daily diets. This review is also believed to be useful for food manufacturer who are interested in producing health foods, utilize new foods resources to make profit, and develop new food resources. This review should also provide very good educational references.

REFERENCES

[1] Rehm J, Samokhvalov AV, Shield KD. Global burden of alcoholic liver diseases. *J. Hepatol.* 2013; 59:160–168.

[2] Wu W, Sun R. Toxicological studies on plant proteins: a review. *J. Appl. Toxicol.* 2011; 32: 377–386.

[3] Wu W, Sun Y. Dietary safety evaluation of water hyacinth leaf protein concentrate. *Hum. Exp. Toxicol.* 2011; 30: 1514–1520.

[4] Williams R. Global Challenges in Liver Disease. *Hepatol.* 2006; 44:521-526.

[5] Wu W, Guo X, Huang M. Evaluation of acute toxicity potential of water hyacinth leaves. *Toxicol. Ind. Health.* 2014; 30(5): 426-431.

[6] Wu W. Dietary Risk Factors of Cardiovascular Diseases. New York: Nova Science Publishers, INC; 2015. ISBN: 978-1-63482-761-4.

[7] Wilkins T, Tadkod A, Hepburn I, Schade RR. Nonalcoholic Fatty Liver Disease: Diagnosis and Management. *Am. Fam. Physician.* 2013; 88(1):35-42.

[8] Bellentani S, Scaglioni F, Marino M, Bedogni G. Epidemiology of non-alcoholic fatty liver disease. *Dig. Dis.* 2010; 28(1):155-161.

[9] Ratziu V, Bellentani S, Cortez-Pinto H, Day C, Marchesini G. A position statement on NAFLD/NASH based on the EASL 2009 special confer-ence. *J. Hepatol.* 2010; 53(2):372-384.

[10] Speliotes EK, Massaro JM, Hoffmann U, Vasan RS, Meigs JB, Sahani DV, et al. Fatty liver is associated with dyslipidemia and dysglycemia independent of visceral fat: the Framingham Heart Study. *Hepatol.* 2010; 51(6):1979-1987.

[11] Angulo P. GI epidemiology: nonalcoholic fatty liver disease. *Aliment Pharmacol. Ther.* 2007; 25(8):883-889.

[12] Loria P, Adinolfi LE, Bellentani S, Bugianesi E, Grieco A, Fargion S, et al. NAFLD Expert Committee of the Associazione Italiana per lo studio del Fegato. Practice guidelines for the diagnosis and management of nonalcoholic fatty liver disease. A decalogue from the Italian Association for the Study of the Liver (AISF) Expert Committee. *Dig. Liver Dis.* 2010; 42(4):272-282.

[13] Lazo M, Hernaez R, Bonekamp S, Kamel IR, Brancati FL, Guallar E, et al. Non-alcoholic fatty liver disease and mortality among US adults: prospective cohort study. *BMJ.* 2011; 343:d6891.

[14] Marra F, Gastaldelli A, Svegliati Baroni G, Tell G, Tiribelli C. Molecular basis and mechanisms of progression of non-alcoholic steatohepatitis. *Trends Mol. Med.* 2008; 14(2):72-81.

[15] Day CP, James OF. Hepatic steatosis: innocent bystander or guilty party? *Hepatol.* 1998; 27(6):1463-1466.

[16] Silvaa M, Gomes S, Peixoto A, Torres-Ramalhoc P, Cardosoa H, Azevedod R, et al. Nutrition in Chronic Liver Disease. *Port J. Gastroenterol.* 2015; http://dx.doi.org/10.1016/j.jpge.2015.06.004.

[17] Rush B. An inquiry into the effects of ardent spirits upon the human body and mind: with an account of the means of preventing, and of the remedies for curing them. 8th ed. Exeter (NH): Richardson; 1785, Reprint.

[18] Rehm J, Shield KD, Rehm MX, Gmel Jr G, Frick U. Alcohol consumption, alcohol dependence, and attributable burden of disease in Europe: potential gains from effective interventions for alcohol dependence. Toronto, Canada: Centre for Addiction and Mental Health; 2012.

[19] NHMRC. Australian guidelines to reduce health risks from drinking alcohol. Canberra ACT 2600, Australia: NHMRC publications; 2009. ISBN Print: 1864963743, ISBN Online: 1864963808.

[20] OECD SIDS. ETHANOL: CAS N: 64-17-5. SIDS Initial Assessment Report For SIAM 19. Berlin, Germany: UNEP PUBLICATIONS; 2004.

[21] Bashir RM, Lewis JH. Hepatotoxicity of drugs used in the treatment of gastrointestinal disorders. *Gastroenterol. Clin. N. Am.* 1995; 24: 937-67.

[22] Kowalski TE, Falestiny M, Furth E, Malet PF. Vitamin A hepatotoxicity: a cautionary note regarding 25,000 IU supplements. *Am. J. Med.* 1994; 97(6):523-8.

[23] Forouhar F, Nadel MS, Gondos B. Hepatic Pathology in Vitamin A Toxicity. *Ann. Clin. Lab. Sci.* 14(4): 304-310.

[24] Penniston KL, Tanumihardjo SA. The acute and chronic toxic effects of vitamin A. *Am. J. Clin. Nutr.* 2006; 83:191–201.

[25] Dietary Reference Intakes for Vitamin A, Vitamin K, Arsenic, Boron, Chromium, Copper, Iodine, Iron, Manganese, Molybdenum, Nickel, Silicon, Vanadium, and Zinc. Washington DC: National Academy Press; 2001. ISBN 0-309-07279-4.

[26] Knip M, Douek IF, Moore WP, Gillmor HA, McLean AE, Bingley PJ, et al. Safety of high-dose nicotinamide: a review. *Diabetologia* 2000; 43(11): 1337–45(2000).

[27] Winter SL, Boyer JL. Hepatic toxicity from large doses of vitamin B_3 (nicotinamide). *N. Engl. J. Med.* 1973; 289:1180-1182.

[28] Gallagher CH, Simmonds RA. Prophylaxis of poisoning by carbon tetrachloride. *Nature* 1959; 184:1407-1408.

[29] Dietary Reference Intakes for Thiamin, Riboflavin, Niacin, Vitamin B_6, Folate, Vitamin B_{12}, Pantothenic Acid, Biotin, and Choline. Washington DC: National Academy Press; 1998. ISBN: 0-309-59725-0.

[30] USDA. Foods list, national nutrient database for standard reference Release 26, 2014. Available at: http://ndb.nal.usda.gov/ndb/foods/show/3834?fg=Beef+Products&man=&lfacet=&format=&count=&max=25& offset=&sort=&qlookup=spleen. Accessed 22 August 2014.

[31] Garg R, Malinow M, Pettinger M, Upson B, Hunninghake D. Niacin treatment increases plasma homocysteine levels. *Am. Heart J.* 1999; 138:1082-1087.

[32] Britton RS, Leicester KL, Bacon BR. Iron Toxicity and Chelation Therapy. *Intern J Hematol.* 2002; 76:219-228.

[33] Piperno A. Classification and diagnosis of iron overload. *Haematol.* 1998; 83:447-455.

[34] Porter JB. Practical management of iron overload. *Br. J. Haematol.* 2001; 115:239-252.

[35] Finch C, Huebers H. Perspectives in iron metabolism. *N. Engl. J. Med.* 1982; 306:1520-8.

[36] Whitlock EP, Garlitz BA, Harris EL, Beil TL, Smith PR. Screening for hereditary hemochromatosis: a systematic review for the U.S. Preventive Services Task Force. *Ann. Intern. Med.* 2006; 145:209-23.

[37] Bouaziz H, Ketata S, Jammoussi K, Boudawara T, Ayedi F, Ellouze F, et al. Effects of sodium fluoride on hepatic toxicity in adult mice and their suckling pups. *Pestic Biochem. Physiol.* 2006; 86(3):124–130.

[38] Parihar S, Choudhary A, Gaur S. Toxicity of fluoride in liver of Albino rat and Mitigation after adopting artificial (Vitamin C and D) and natural (Aloe vera) food supplementations. *Intern J. Adv. Res. Technol.* 2013; 2(2):1-11.

[39] Yang K, Liang X. Fluoride in Drinking Water: Effect on Liver and Kidney Function. *Encyclopedia of Enviromental Health*, 2011. p. 179-775.

[40] Dietary Reference Intakes for Calcium, Phosphorus, Magnesium, Vitamin D, and Fluoride. Washington DC: National Academy Press; 1997. ISBN 0-309-06350-7 (cloth). — ISBN 0-309-06403-1 (pbk).

[41] Opinion of the Scientific Panel on Contaminants in the Food Chain on a request of the Commission related to concentration limits for boron and fluoride in natural mineral waters (Question N° EFSA-Q-2003-21). *EFSA. J.* 2005; 237:1-8.

[42] Al-Bader A, Abul H, Hussain T, Al-Moosawi M, Mathew TC, Dashti H. Selenium and liver cirrhosis. *Mol. Cell Biochem.* 1998; 185(1-2):1-6.

[43] Aaseth J, Smith-Kielland A, Thomassen Y. Selenium, alcohol and liver diseases. *Ann. Clin. Res.* 1986; 18(1):43-7.

[44] Thuluvath PJ, Triqer DR. Selenium in chronic liver disease. *J. Hepatol.* 1992; 14(2-3): 176-182.

[45] Nuttall KL. Review: Evaluating Selenium Poisoning. *Ann. Clin. Lab. Sci.* 2006; 36(4): 409-420.

[46] Dridietary Reference Intakes for Vitamin C, Vitamin E, Selenium, and Carotenoids. Washington DC: National Academy Press; 2000. ISBN 0-309-06949-1 (case) -- ISBN 0-309-06935-1 (paper).

[47] Hagan EC, Jenner PM, Jones WI, Fitzhugh OG, Long EL, Brouwer JG, et al. Toxic properties of compounds related to safrole. *Toxicol. Appl. Pharmacol.* 1965; 7:18-24.

[48] Miller EC, Swanson AB, Phillips DH, Fetcher TL, Liem A, Miller JA. Structure-activity studies of the carcinogenicities in the mouse and rat of some naturally occurring and synthetic alkenylbenzene derives related to safrole and estragole. *Cancer Res.* 1983; 43:1124-1134.

[49] Jin M, Kijima A, Suzuki Y, Hibi D, Inoue T, Ishii Y, et al. Comprehensive toxicity study of safrole using a medium-term animal model with gpt delta rats. *Toxicol.* 2011; 290(2-3):312-21.

[50] Liu TY, Chen CC, Chen CL, Chi CW. Safrole-induced Oxidative Damage in the Liver of Sprague-Dawley Rats. *Food Chem. Toxicol.* 1999; 37(7):697-702.

[51] European Commission, Scientific Committee on Food (SCF). Opinion of the Scientific Committee on Food on the safety of the presence of safrole (1-allyl-3,4-methylene dioxy benzene) in flavourings and other food ingredients with flavouring properties. http://ec.europa.eu/food/fs/sc/scf/out116_en.pdf (2001; Accessed 20 August 2015).

[52] Da Silva Negreiros JR, Miqueloni DP, Da Cunha Cartaxo CB. Yield of essential oil and safrole content based on fresh and dry biomass of long pepper in the Brazilian Amazon. *Acta Amazonica* 2015; 45(1):75 – 80.

[53] Agrawal RC, Bhide SV. Histopathological studies on toxicity of Chilli (Capsaicin) in Syrian golden hamsters. *Indian J. Experim. Biol.* 1988; 26:377-382.
[54] Hoch-Ligeti C. Production of liver tumours bydietary means: Effect of feeding chillies to rats. *Acta Unio Internationalis Contra Cancrum* 1951; 7:606-611.
[55] European Commission, Scientific Committee on Food (SCF). Opinion of the Scientific Committee on Food on Capsaicin (adopted on 26 February 2002). http://ec.europa.eu/food/fs/sc/scf/out120_en.pdf (2002; Accessed 25 August 2015).
[56] Glinsukon T, Stitmunnaithum V, Toskulkao C, Buranawuti T, Tangkrisanavinont V. Acute toxicity of capsaicin in several animal species. *Toxicon* 1980; 18:215-220.
[57] Monsereenusorn Y, Kongsamut S, Pezalla PD. Capsaicin-a literature survey. *Crit. Rev. Toxicol.* 1982; 10:321–339.
[58] Monsereenusorn Y. Subchronic toxicity studies of capsaicin and capsicum in rats. *Res. Commun. Chem. Pathol. Pharmacol.* 1983; 41(1):95-110.
[59] Jang JJ, Devor DE, Logsdon DL, Ward JM. A 4-week feeding study of ground red chilli (Capsicum annuum) in male B6C3F1 mice. *Food Chem. Toxicol.* 1992; 30:783-787.
[60] Lee SO. Studies on the influence of diets and lipotropic substances upon the various organs and metabolic changes in rabbits on long term feeding with red pepper. *Korean J. Intern. Med.* 1963; 6(7):383-395.
[61] Surh YJ, Lee SS. Capsaicin, A Double-Edged Sword: Toxicity, Metabolism, and Chemopreventive Poential. *Life Sci.* 1995, 56(22):1845-1855.
[62] Parrish M. Liquid chromatographic method of determining capsaicinoids in capsicumsand their extractives: Collaborative study. *J. Assoc. Off Anal. Chem. Intern.* 1996; 79(3):738-745.
[63] Thomas BV. Schreiber AA, Weisskopf CP. Simple method for quantitation of capsaicinoids in peppers using capillary gas chromatography. *J Agric. Food Chem.* 1998; 46:2655-2663.
[64] Lopez-Hernandez J, Oruna-Concha MJ, Simal-Lozano J, Gonzales-Castro MJ, Vazquez-Blanco ME. Determination of capsaicin and dihydrocapsaicin in cayenne pepper and padron peppers by HPLC. *Deutsche Lebensmittel-Rundschau* 1996; 92:393-395.
[65] Bergmann K. Expert Report on the Assessmentof Coumarin in Medicinal Products with regard to Hepatotoxic Effects in Humans. Bonn: Rheinische Friedrich-Wilhelms-Universität; 1999.
[66] Norwegian Scientific Committee for Food Safety. Risk assessment of coumarin intake in the Norwegianpopulation: Opinion of the Panel on Food Additives, Flavourings, Processing Aids, *Materials in Contact with Food and Cosmetics of the Norwegian Scientific Committee for Food Safety*, 13 October 2010. ISBN 978-82-8259-005 1.
[67] Coumarin in flavourings and other food ingredients with flavouring properties: Scientific Opinion of the Panel onFood Additives, Flavourings, Processing Aids and Materials in Contact with Food (AFC) (Question No EFSA-Q-2008-677). *EFSA. J.* 2008; 793:1-15.
[68] Beinssen APC. Possible coumarin hepatotoxicity. *Med. J. Australia.* 1994; 161:725.
[69] Casley-Smith JR, Casley-Smith JR. Frequency of coumarin hepatotoxicity. *Medical J. Australia.* 1995; 162:391.

[70] Morrison L, Welsby PD. Side-effects of coumarin. *Postgrad. Med. J.* 1995; 71:701 – 702.

[71] Basset ML, Dahlström JE. Liver Failure while taking coumarin. *Med. J. Australia.* 1995; 163:106.

[72] Koch S, Beurton I, Bresson-Hadni S, Monnot B, Hrusovsky S, Becker M, et al. Acute cytolytic hepatitis caused by coumarin. Two cases. *Gastroenterol Clin. Biol.* 1997; 21:223-225.

[73] Lake BG, Gray TJB, Evans JG, Lewis*DFV, Beamand JA, Hue KL. Studies on the mechanism of coumarin-induced toxicity in rat hepatocytes: Comparison with dihydrocoumarin and other coumarin metabolites. *Toxicol. Appl. Pharmacol.* 1989; 97(2):311–323.

[74] Risk assessment of coumarin intake in the Norwegian population: Opinion of the Panel on Food Additives, Flavourings, Processing Aids, *Materials in Contact with Food and Cosmetics of theNorwegian Scientific Committee for Food Safety*, 13 October 2010. ISBN 978-82-8259-005-1.

[75] BfR (Federal Institute for Risk Assessment). Consumers, who eat a lot of cinnamon, currently have an overly high exposure to coumarin. BfR Health Assessment No. 043/2006, 16 June 2006.

[76] Kakani R, Gamboa DA, Calhoun MC, Haq AU, Bailey CA. Relative toxicity of cottonseed gossypol enantiomers in broilers. *Open Toxicol. J.* 2010; 4:26–31.

[77] Blevins S, Siegel PB, Blodgett DJ, Ehrich M, Saunders GK, Lewis RM. Effects of silymarin on gossypol toxicosis in divergent lines of chickens. *Poultry Sci.* 2010; 89(9):1878–1886.

[78] Deoras DP, Young-Curtis P, Dalvi RR, Tippett FE. Effect of gossypol on hepatic and serum γ-glutamyltransferase activity in rats. *Vet. Res. Commun.* 1997; 21(5):317–323.

[79] Fonseca NBS, Gadelha ICN, Oloris SCS, Soto-Blanco B. Effectiveness of albumin-conjugated gossypol as an immunogen to prevent gossypol-associated acute hepatotoxicity in rats. *Food Chem. Toxicol.* 2013; 56:149–153.

[80] El-Sharaky AS, Newairy AA, Elguindy NM, Elwafa AA. Spermatotoxicity, biochemical changes and histological alteration induced by gossypol in testicular and hepatic tissues of male rats. *Food Chem. Toxicol.* 2010; 48(12):3354–3361.

[81] Wang Y, Lei HP. Hepatotoxicity of gossypol in rats. *J. Ethnopharmacol.* 1987; 20(1):53–64.

[82] Manabe S, Nuber DC, Lin YC. Zone-specific hepatotoxicity of gossypol in perfused rat liver. *Toxicon* 1991; 29(6):787–790.

[83] Gadelha ICN, Fonseca NBS, Oloris SCS, Melo MM, Soto-Blanco B. Gossypol Toxicity from Cottonseed Products. *Sci. World J.* 2014; 2014:Article ID 231635, 11 pages. http://dx.doi.org/10.1155/2014/231635.

[84] Luís de Carvalho W, Maioli MA, Mendes LCN, Rozza DB, Mingatto FE. Mechanisms of the intoxication of rat liver caused by gossypol. *Pesq. Vet. Bras.* 2013; 33(3):339-344.

[85] Gossypol as undesirable substance in animal feed: Scientific Opinion of the Panel on Contaminants in the Food Chain (Question No EFSA-Q-2005-222). *EFSA J.* 2008; 908:1-55.

[86] Percy RG, Calhoun MC, Kim HL. Seed gossypol variation within Gossypium barbadense L. cotton. *Crop Sci.* 1996; 36(1):193–197.

[87] Calhoun MC, Kuhlmann SK, Balwin BC. Assessing the gossypol status of cattle fed cotton feed products. *Proceedings of the Pacific Northwest Animal Nutrition Conference*, 1995. p. 147A–158A.

[88] Stipanovic RD, Puckhaber LS, Liu J, Bell AA. Total and percent atropisomers of Gossypol and Gossypol-6-methyl ether in seeds from Pima cottons and accessions of Gossypium barbadense L. *J. Agric. Food Chem.* 2009; 57(2):566–571.

[89] Scientific Opinion on Pyrrolizidine alkaloids in food and feed. *EFSA J.* 2011; 9(11):2406.

[90] NTP (National Toxicology Program). NTP technical report on toxicity studies of riddelliine. NTP Toxicity Report Series, Number 27, 1992.

[91] Chan PC, Haseman JK, Prejean JD, Nyska A. Toxicity and carcinogenicity of riddelliine in rats and mice. *Toxicol. Lett.* 2003; 144:295-311.

[92] Cheeke PR. Toxicity and metabolism of pyrrolizidine alkaloids. *J. Anim. Sci.* 1988; 66(9):2343-50.

[93] Dübecke A, Beckh G, Lüllmann C. Pyrrolizidine Alkaloids in honey and pollen. *Food Add Contamin.* 2011; 28:348-358.

[94] Fu PP, Yang YC, Xia Q, Chou MW, Cui YY, Lin G. Pyrrolizidine alkaloids – Tumorigenic components in Chinese herbal medicines and dietary supplements. *J. Food Drug Analys.* 2002; 10:198-211.

[95] Sieber SM, Correa P, Dalgard DW, McIntire KR, Adamson RH. Carcinogenicity and Hepatotoxicity of Cycasin and Its Aglycone Methylazoxymethanol Acetate in Nonhuman Primates. *JNCI J. Natl. Cancer Inst.* 1980; 65(1):177-189.

[96] Williams PD, Murphy GP. Dose related effects of cycasin induced renal and hepatic tumors. *Res. Commun. Chem. Pathol. Pharmacol.* 1971; 2(4):627-32.

[97] Dooley KL, Von Tungeln LS, Bucci T, Fu PP, Kadlubar FF. Comparative carcinogenicity of 4-aminobiphenyl and the food pyrolysates, Glu-P-1, IQ, PhIP, and MeIQx in the neonatal B6C3F1male mouse. *Cancer Lett.* 1992; 62:205-209.

[98] NTP. Report on Carcinogens Background Document for Heterocyclic Amines: PhIP, MeIQ and MeIQx. National Toxicology Program; 2002. Available from: http://ntp.niehs.nih.gov/ntp/newhomeroc/roc11/HCAs Pub.pdf.

[99] Ushijima T, Makino H, Kakiuchi H, Inoue R, Sugimura T, Nagao M. Genetic alterations in HCA-induced tumors. *Princess Takamatsu Symp.* 1995; 23:281-291.

[100] Von Tungeln LS, Bucci TJ, Hart RW, Kadlubar FF, Fu PP. Inhibitory effect of caloric restriction on tumorigenicity induced by 4-aminobiphenyl and 2-amino-1-methyl-6-phenylimidazo-[4,5-b]pyridine (PhIP) in the CD1 newborn mouse bioassay. *Cancer Lett.* 1996; 104:133-136.

[101] Dass SB, Bucci TJ, Heflich RH, Casciano DA. Evaluation of the transgenic p53+/- mouse for detecting genotoxic liver carcinogens in a short-term bioassay. *Cancer Lett.* 1999; 43:81-85.

[102] Eisenbrand G, Tang W. Food-borneheterocyclic amines: Chemistry, formation, occurrences and biological activities: A literature review. *Toxicol.* 1993; 84:1-82.

[103] Cross AJ, Sinha R. Meat-related mutagens/carcinogens in the etiology of colorectal cancer. *Environ. Molec. Mutag.* 2004; 44(1):44–55.

[104] Robbana-Barnat S, Rabache M, Rialland E, Fradin J. Heterocyclic Amines: Occurrence and Prevention in Cooked Food. *Environ. Health Perspect.* 1996; 104:280-288.

[105] Jägerstad M, Skog K. Genotoxicity of heat-processed foods. *Mutat. Res.* 2005; 574(1–2):156–172.
[106] Suqimura T, Wakabayashi K, Nakagama H, Nagao M. Heterocyclic amines: Mutagenns/carcinogens produced during cooking of meat and fish. *Cancer Sci.* 2004; 95(4):290-299.
[107] Haun CC, Kinkead ER. Chronic inhalation toxicity of hydrazine. Proceedings of the 4th Annual Conference on Environmental Toxicology. *Wright-Patterson Air Force Base*, OH; 1973. AMRL-TR-73-125:351-363.
[108] Comstock CC, Lawson LH, Greene EA, Oberst FW. Inhalation toxicity of hydrazine vapor. *Arch. Ind. Hyg. Occup. Med.* 1954; 10:476-490.
[109] Sotaniemi E, Hivonen J, Isomaki H, Takkunen J, Kaila J. Hydrazine toxicity in the human. Report of a fatal case. *Ann. Clin. Res.* 1971; 3:30-33.
[110] Selim K, Kaplowitz A. Hepatotoxicity of Psychotropic Drugs. *Hepatol.* 1999; 29(5):1347-1351.
[111] Nagaoka MH, Nagaoka H, Kondo K, Akiyama H, Maitani T. Measurement of a Genotoxic Hydrazine, Agaritine, and Its Derivatives by HPLC with Fluorescence Derivatization in the Agaricus Mushroom and Its Products. *Chem. Pharm. Bull.* 2006; 54(6):922—924.
[112] Hashida C, Hayashi K, Jie L, Haga S, Sakurai M, Shimizu H. Quantities of agaritine in mushrooms (Agaricus bisporus) and the carcinogenicity of mushroom methanol extracts on the mouse bladder epithelium. *Nippon Koshu Eisei Zasshi.* 1990; 37(6):400–405.
[113] Larsson B, Eriksson A. The analysis and occurrence of hydrazine toxins in fresh and processed false morel, Gyromitra esculenta. *Zeitschrift für Lebensmittel-Untersuchung und -Forschung* 1989; 189(5):438-442.
[114] Teschke R, Qiu SX, Xuan TD, Lebot V. Kava and Kava Hepatotoxicity: Requirements for Novel Experimental, Ethnobotanical and Clinical Studies Based on a Review of the Evidence. *Phytother Res.* 2011; 25:1263–1274.
[115] Brauer RB, Pfab R, Becker K, Berger H, Stangl M. Fulminantes leberversagen nach einnahme des pflazlichen heilmittels kava-kava. *Z. Gastroenterol.* 2001; 39:491.
[116] Escher M, Desmeules J, Giostra E, Mentha G. Hepatitis associated with kava, a herbal remedy for anxiety. *BMJ.* 2001; 322(7279):139.
[117] Kraft M, Spahn TW, Menzel J, Senninger N, Dietl KH, Herbst H, et al. Fulminant liver failure after administration of the herbal antidepressant kava-kava. *Dtsch. Med. Wochenschr.* 2001; 126(36):970-972.
[118] Saß M, Schnabel S, Kröger J, Liebe S, Schareck WD. Acute liver failure from kava-kava-a rare indication for liver transplantation. *Z. Gastroenterol.* 2001;39:491.
[119] Campo JV, McNabb J, Perel JM, Mazariegos GV, Hasegawa SL, Reyes J. Kava-induced fulminant hepatic failure. *J. Am. Acad. Child Adolesc. Psych.* 2002; 41:631-632.
[120] Humbertston C, Akhtar J, Krenzelok E. Acute hepatitis induced by kava kava, an herbal product derived from *Piper methysticum*. *J. Clin. Toxicol.* 2001; 39:549.
[121] Russmann S, Lauterburg BH, Helbling A. Kava hepatotoxicity. *Ann. Intern. Med.* 2001; 135:68-69.

[122] Food and Drug Administration. Letter to health-care professionals: FDA issues consumer advisory that kava products may be associated with severe liver injury. Rockville, Maryland: U.S. Department of Health and Human Services, Food and Drug Administration, 2002. Available at http://www.cfsan.fda.gov/~dms/addskava.html.

[123] Connor KM, Davidson JRT, Churchill LE. Adverse effect profile of kava. *CNS Spectr.* 2001; 6:848-853.

[124] Singh YN. Kava: an overview. *J. Ethnopharmacol.* 1992; 37:13-45.

[125] Lebot V, Merlin M, Lindstom L. Kava the Pacific Drug. Newhaven: Yale University Press; 1992. p. 255.

[126] SCF (Scientific Committee on Food). Opinion of the Scientific Committee on Food on pulegone and 598 menthofuran. SCF/CS/FLAV/FLAVOUR/3 ADD2 Final 25 July 2002.

[127] NTP. Toxicology and carcinogenesis 591studies of pulegone (CAS No. 89-82-7) in F344/N rats and B6C3F1 mice (gavage studies). *Natl Toxicol Program Tech. Rep Ser.* 2011; 2011(563):1-201.

[128] EFSA. STUDY on the Assessment of Plants/Herbs, Plant/Herb Extracts And Their Naturally Or Synthetically Produced Components As "Additives" For Use In Animal Production CFT/EFSA/FEEDAP/2005/01. Available at http://www.efsa.europa.eu/sites/default/files/scientific_ output/files/main_documents/070828.pdf.

[129] Wang Jb, Zhao HP, Zhao YI, Jin C, Liu DJ, Kong WJ, et al. Hepatotoxicity or Hepatoprotection? Pattern Recognition for the Paradoxical Effect of the Chinese Herb Rheum palmatum L. in Treating Rat Liver Injury. *PLoS ONE* 2011; 6(9):e24498.

[130] Murdiati TB, McSweeney CS, Campbell RS, Stoltz DS. Prevention of hydrolysable tannin toxicity in goats fed Clidemia hirta by calcium hydroxide supplementation. *J. Appl. Toxicol.* 1990; 10:325–331.

[131] Sathaye S, Bagul Y, Gupta S, Kaur H, Redkar R. Hepatoprotective effects of aqueous leaf extract and crude isolates of Murraya koenigii against in vitro ethanol-induced hepatotoxicity model. *Exp. Toxicol. Pathol.* 2011; 63(6):587-91.

[132] EFSA. Scientific opinion on saponins in Madhuca longifolia L. as undesirable substances in animal feed. *EFSA. J.* 2009; 979:1-36.

[133] Sharma OP, Sharma S, Pattabhi V, Mahato SB, Sharma PD. *Crit. Rev. Toxicol.* 2007; 37(4):313-52.

[134] Güçlü-Üstünda Ö, Mazza G. Saponins: Properties, applications and processing. *Cr. Rev. Food Sci. Nutr.* 2007; 47:231-258(2007).

[135] Ilsley SE, Miller HM, Kamel C. Effects of dietary Quillajasaponin and curcumin on the performance and immune status of weaned piglets. *J. Anim. Sci.* 2005; 83:82-88.

[136] Turner JL, Dritz SS, Higgins JJ, Herkelman KL, Minton JE. Effects of a Quillaja saponariaextract on growth performance and immune function of weanling pigs challenged with Salmonella typhimurium. *J. Anim. Sci.* 2002; 80:1939-1946.

[137] Qin Y, Wu X, Huang W, Gong G, Li D, He Y, et al. Acute toxicity and sub-chronic toxicity of steroidal saponins from Dioscorea zingiberensis C. H. Wright in rodents. *J. Ethnopharmacol.* 2009; 126(3):543-50.

[138] Güçlü-Üstündag Ö, Mazza G. Saponins: Properties, applications and processing. *Cr. Rev. Food Sci. Nutr.* 2007; 47:231-258.

[139] Ireland PA, Dziedzic SZ, Kearsley MW. Saponin content of soya and some commercial soya products by means of high-performance liquid-chromatography of the sapogenins. *J. Sci. Food Agric.* 1986; 37(7):694-698.

[140] Knudsen D, Ron O, Baardsen G, Smedsgaard J, Koppe W, Frokiaer H. Soyasaponins resist extrusion cooking and are notdegraded during gut passage in Atlantic salmon (Salmo salarL.). *J. Agric. Food Chem.* 2006; 54:6428-6435.

In: Diets and Diseases: Causes and Prevention
Editor: Wenbiao Wu

ISBN: 978-1-63484-580-9

Chapter 6

DIET AND LIVER DISEASES: CAUSES, PREVENTION AND DIETARY MANAGEMENT

Oluwatoyin Bolanle Oluwole*, Elemo Olubunmi, Olasehinde Oluwatosin and Adesioye Temiloluwa
Department of Food Technology,
Federal Institute of Industrial Research, Oshodi, Lagos, Nigeria

ABSTRACT

The liver is the most complex and largest internal organ in the human body. It plays an important role in the proper functioning of internal environment through its multiple and diverse functions. The liver is prone to a number of diseases as a result of its multidimensional function. The diseases are categorized into chronic and acute liver diseases. The burden of chronic liver disease is increasing in both developed as well as developing countries. The main cause for this continuous rise of liver disease is non-alcoholic fatty liver disease (NAFLD). Hepatitis, another form of liver disease is also affecting millions of people worldwide. Though, it is possible for an individual to survive with 70% liver damage, there is a substantial problem in the number of death arising from liver disease. This causes a high cost to nations in the sector of health. Thus, this generally causes a huge economic burden to the nation at large.

Diet plays significant roles in the management or development of liver disease. Polyunsaturated fatty acid, proteins and minerals are important requirements in patient suffering from certain liver diseases. However, there are certain dietary related factors causing liver diseases such as obesity, protein-energy malnutrition, vitamin toxicity and aflatoxin exposure. Diet has also been found to confer hepatoprotective effect on the liver from various studies especially diet high in antioxidant content, as several liver diseases are associated with oxidative stress. However despite these possibilities, antioxidants have produced different results in various studies, as some have reported efficacy in treating liver disease while others have not. However, dietary fatty acid has also been found to play an important role in the pathogenesis of liver disease.

* Corresponding Author address: Department of Food Technology, Federal Institute of Industrial Research, Oshodi, Lagos, Nigeria. Email: oluwatoyinoluwole575@yahoo.com.

Consequently in this chapter, the causes and prevalence of different liver diseases are discussed, the role of consuming food grains with high level of aflatoxin in the etiology of liver diseases and appropriate diet for prevention as part of management strategies of the different liver diseases are discussed.

Food industries are therefore urged to develop and produce appropriate nutritious food products for this category of the populace. In addition, food products meant for public consumption should be such that will not pose health risk such as for both acute and chronic liver diseases.

INTRODUCTION

The liver is an important internal organ in the body. It weighs about 1.44–1.66 kg (3.2–3.7 lb) and as such, suggested to be the largest internal organ in the human body [1]. The liver is reddish brown and triangular in shape. It is located in the right upper quadrant of the abdominal cavity where it lies attached to the diaphragm, to the right of the stomach and overlying the gallbladder. The liver has highly specialized tissue consisting of mostly hepatocytes (liver cells) which regulates a wide variety of high-volume biochemical reactions, including the synthesis and breakdown of small and complex molecules, many of which are necessary for normal vital functions [2].

The liver is the only human internal organ capable of naturally regenerating its lost tissue. It has been discovered that 25% of the liver is capable of regenerating into a whole liver [3]. However, it is important to note that the regeneration or growth of the liver involves restoration of function and not structure. Thus exact structure may not necessarily be restored. The liver functions through deriving its blood supply from hepatic portal veins and hepatic arteries. Hepatic portal vein carries venous blood drained from the spleen, gastrointestinal tract, and its associated organ, this enables the liver to be the first organ to encounter ingested nutrients, drugs and environmental toxicants that enter the hepatic portal vein from the digestive system [4].

The history relating to liver regeneration, can be traced back to Greek mythology where Prometheus was punished by the gods for revealing fire to humans, by being chained to a rock where a vulture would peck out his liver, which would regenerate overnight. “Hepar” is the Greek term for liver, which has become the term synonymous to liver related medical terms starting with, “hepatic” or “hepato.” The Greeks considered the liver to be the home of all human emotions. It was thought to be the seat of the darkest emotions (specifically wrath, jealousy and greed) which drove men to action [5].

FUNCTIONS OF THE LIVER

The liver plays an important role in the maintenance of internal environment through its multiple and diverse functions [6]. Some of the functions include: protein synthesis (amino acid, albumin, hormones and blood clotting factors), fatty acid and cholesterol synthesis, metabolism and storage of carbohydrates, formation and secretion of bile, degradation of red blood cell, metabolism of exogenous compound and the production of biochemicals necessary for digestion. The liver breaks down or modifies toxic substances and medicinal products in a process called drug metabolism. This sometimes results in intoxication, when the metabolite is more toxic than its precursor. Preferably, the toxins are conjugated to avail excretion in bile or urine. In the fetus, the liver does not perform usual functions but rather is involved in the formation of blood stem cells and releases them to the fetal thymus [7]. The formation of blood stem cells shifts to the red bone marrow after birth. Several other functions are performed by the liver. The liver is responsible for up to 500 separate functions, usually in combination with other systems and organs [8].

ROLE OF THE LIVER IN NUTRITION

Food is a complex, heterogeneous mixture of vastly numerous and diverse biochemical substances [9]. Food is broken down in the stomach and small intestine to produce small water soluble food molecules or nutrients. The food molecules are absorbed through the small intestine into the blood stream and transported to the liver where the food molecules are either stored or broken down further to be readily used by the body depending on the needs of the body at that period.

Food contains primarily carbohydrate, fat and protein as the three main sources of energy and they comprise 90% of the dry weight of food [10]. Carbohydrate and fat are the actual main sources of energy while protein is used for growth and repair of the body. The liver plays an important role in the synthesis, metabolism, secretion and storage of carbohydrate, protein and fats [11]. The liver also stores vitamins (vitamin A, vitamin D, vitamin B_{12}, vitamin K) [12] and minerals (iron, and copper).

Carbohydrate in the diet is mostly derived from starch and sugar. It is found more often in sweet or starchy foods. Carbohydrate is broken down in the liver to glucose. When glucose is not needed for an immediate supply of energy, it is stored as glycogen in the liver and muscles. The liver then degrades the glycogen into glucose when the body requires immediate energy supply. The liver also plays an important role in the regulation of glucose in the blood [13]. It is also capable of synthesizing glucose from certain amino acids, lactate or glycerol.

Protein in the diet is derived from animal sources and plant sources. Protein is made up of units called amino acid. In the liver they provide the necessary building blocks to synthesize hormones, protein carriers (albumin, globulin) cells (red blood cell, white blood cell), platelets and other important tissues in the body. The liver is also responsible for protein metabolism and degradation [14].

Fat in the diet is also derived from plant sources and animal sources. Fat is digested with bile, an alkaline compound produced by the liver. The bile aids in the digestion of fat via the emulsification of lipids and helps in the absorption of vitamin A, D, E and K from the diet. Some of the bile drain directly into the duodenum, and some are stored in the gallbladder. The fat can also be stored in form of triglycerides, as long term energy reserve in the liver. The liver performs several other roles in lipid metabolism [15]. It is involved in cholesterol and lipoprotein synthesis.

LIVER DISEASES

The multidimensional function of the liver makes it prone to various diseases. The burden of chronic liver diseases is on the increase in both developed as well as developing countries. These diseases interfere with liver function and leads to its derangement. However, the liver has a great reserve capacity to regenerate and it only produces symptoms after extensive damage. There are various forms of liver diseases. They are categorized into chronic and acute diseases. Acute diseases occur rapidly and exist for a short period while chronic liver diseases involve a process of progressive destruction and regeneration of liver parenchyma leading to fibrosis and cirrhosis [16]. The non-alcoholic fatty liver disease (NAFLD) is one of the most common forms of chronic liver diseases in the developed world [17]. NAFLD refers to a spectrum of liver disorders occurring due to abnormal fat deposition in the liver from obesity, type 2 diabetes and related metabolic diseases. It ranges in severity from simple hepatic steatosis with no inflammation to steatohepatitis which can progress to liver cirrhosis. NAFLD patients have significant lobular inflammation, hepatocellular necrosis, pericellular and portal fibrosis. Alcohol fatty liver disease (ALD) is also another liver disorder. It has been suggested to be the oldest form of liver damage known to mankind. It is caused by excessive alcohol consumption. However, it is common for patients with ALD to share the risk factors for additional injury from other forms of liver insult such as hepatitis and NAFLD, though patients with fatty liver are initially asymptomatic, so that they rarely present with liver related problems. Fatty liver is reversible with abstention but it is a risk factor for progression to alcoholic hepatitis and cirrhosis in patients who continue drinking [18].

Hepatitis is another common condition of inflammation of the liver. The most usual cause of hepatitis is viral. However, they can also be caused by other factors such as infections, autoimmune diseases, metabolic disorders and toxic substances including alcohol and certain drugs. The most common of the hepatitis infections by virus include: hepatitis A, hepatitis B, hepatitis C, hepatitis D and hepatitis E. Infection with hepatitis B virus or hepatitis C virus has been suggested to be the main cause of liver cancer [19, 20]. The hepatitis A and E occurs through ingestion of contaminated food and water while hepatitis B, C and D occurs as a result of contact with body fluids as seen in sexual transmission. Hepatitis can heal naturally on its own or can progress to fibrosis and cirrhosis, as seen in chronic hepatitis. However, it initially occurs without symptoms but later leads to jaundice and loss of appetite.

Liver cancer is another common form of liver diseases. It manifests as hepatocellular carcinoma or cholangiocarcinoma. Most cases of hepatocellular carcinoma (HC) are found in patients who have been predisposed to other forms of chronic liver diseases and cirrhosis. Necrosis, fibrosis and inflammation also facilitate the development of HC. Hepatitis B virus has also been linked to the development of HC [21]. It is believed that the hepatitis virus may contribute to modify a variety of pathways which may lead to genetic changes (in PIKCA, p53, β–catenin genes) that encourages the development of tumour. Moreover, these liver malignancies could also be secondary lesions that have metastasized from primary cancers in the gastrointestinal tract and other organs, such as the kidney, lungs, breast or prostate. Other diseases of the liver include fascioliasis, cirrhosis, Budd-Chiari syndrome, hereditary associated liver diseases and sclerosing choangitis.

EPIDEMIOLOGY

NAFLD is on the increase worldwide. It is the most common diagnosis in subjects with altered aminotransferases in Western world, where 20-30% of the population is affected [22]. The prevalence of NAFLD in the general population ranges from 10%-24% in various countries. NAFLD affects 40%-75% of patients with type 2 diabetes mellitus, 33%-76% of obese and 90% of morbidly obese people [23]. Moreover, the prevalence of NAFLD among children has increased from 3% to 5% worldwide with 40-70% among obese children [24].

ALD accounts for 37% of liver disease death. It contributes to over 4% of mortality globally. ALD majorly affects the western countries. In 2008, 0.95% of all deaths registered in people aged 20 years and above in United Kingdom was attributed to ALD [25]. Moreover, increased amount of alcohol consumption has been linked to increase ALD. Alcoholic hepatitis, a common and distinct subset of patients with ALD, occurs in 35-40% with chronic excessive alcohol abuse and has a high mortality rate of about 40%-50% in untreated patients with severe diseases [26].

Hepatitis is on the increase globally. Ten million new cases of hepatitis have been reported annually. Hepatitis B virus has an estimate of 350 million people chronically infected [27] and about 170 million people are infected with hepatitis C virus worldwide [28]. Every year 18,000 people have been reported to die due to liver cirrhosis caused by viral hepatitis [29]. Amongst the countries reported to have a high prevalence include Africa, Asian countries (except Japan), America and Eastern European countries. Most of these countries have 5-15% of the population affected chronically with hepatitis B virus. Moreover, it is also reported that a high amount of certain sexual practices has contributed to the prevalence of viral hepatitis in the world.

Primary liver cancer is the fifth most common cancer worldwide, with a wide geographic distribution. It accounts for an estimate of 600,000 deaths annually in the world. In developed countries, such as the United States, it has been linked to approximately 10,000 deaths annually. It is high in East Asia and Sub Saharan Africa (>20 per 100,000) and lower, but on the increase in North America and most of Europe (<5 per 100,000) [30]. One of the major contributors to high incidence of hepatocellular carcinoma in Asia and in Africa is dietary exposure to Aflatoxin [31], which is a common contaminant of foods such as peanuts, grain, legumes and corn. HIV is also thought to increase the rate of liver cancers.

Though people survive with 70% liver damage, there is a substantial burden of morbidity from liver disease, a high cost to the NHS and a huge economic and human cost from liver related ill health. Thus, a high incidence or prevalence of liver diseases is a serious source of concern worldwide.

PATHOGENESIS

The basic pathophysiology of all forms of liver disease represent failures of the numerous and complex hepatic metabolic functions. In NAFLD, defects in fatty acid metabolism are responsible for its pathogenesis. This may be due to imbalance in energy consumption and its combustion, resulting in lipid storage and accumulation of triglycerides in the liver, and this is merely a marker for deranged metabolism and indicates increased lipid trafficking [32]. It can also be a peripheral resistance to insulin, where the transport of fatty acid from adipose tissue to the liver is increased [33]. It has been reported that free fatty acids directly play roles in promoting liver damage by activating inflammatory pathways and increasing oxidative stress leading to toxicity [34].

ALD also has a multifactorial pathology. Energy metabolism, oxidative stress and immunologic mechanisms contribute to the development of alcoholic liver disease. Chronic alcohol consumption depresses the activity of the mitochondrial process. Some of the defects are found in the impaired electron transport, impaired proton translocation, decreased heme content of cytochrome oxidase and reduced function in ATP synthase complex [35]. These factors impair energy metabolism of liver cells and lead to tissue damage. Moreover, ethanol metabolism produces acetaldehyde which forms a hybrid adduct with reactive residues, mediating lipid peroxidation and nucleic acid oxidation [36]. The lipid peroxidation adducts formed are highly toxic to the hepatocytes. They stimulate an increased amount of circulating antibodies in the liver and this results in an impaired immune response as proinflammatory cytokines are increased which facilitates liver tissue damage [37].

The pathophysiology of hepatitis varies and depends on the underlying cause of the condition. In viral hepatitis, the presence of hepatitis virus (A, B, C, D and E) affects the host immune cells as they respond to viral proteins expressed by the infected hepatocytes. This results in the initiation of a cascade of antigen nonspecific effector systems which ends up causing necroinflammatory disease. In auto immune hepatitis, the auto reactive T-cell mediated cascade is directed against the liver antigens occurring in genetically susceptible individuals. However, this may also occur from prior liver damage from environment, drugs or viral infection [38]. Alcoholic hepatitis is caused by the excessive consumption of alcohol. It is suggested that the metabolism of alcohol increases toxic adducts that facilitate the action of endotoxin on kupffer cells which may lead to liver infection [39]. Cytokines and immunity are also actively involved in its pathogenesis.

Liver cancer or hepatocellular carcinoma may arise from multifactorial events. They could be as a result of mutations in the cells regulating apoptosis, causing an increase in cell proliferation. Hepatocellular carcinoma development has also been linked to hepatitis virus and underlying cirrhotic liver disease. The hepatitis virus may stimulate the host immune response to attack the liver cells which might result into a cycle of repair. The defects found in repair pathway may degenerate into carcinogenesis. Alcohol has also been suggested to play a role in liver cancer by integrating defects in the genome of infected cells arising from predisposition to endotoxins. Another contributing factor to hepatocellular carcinoma is aflatoxins. Aflatoxin from aspergillus species has been shown to cause hepatocellular carcinoma with continuous build up in the liver [40].

Management

In managing alcoholic and non- alcoholic fatty liver diseases, the most effective system adopted involves making life style changes such as cutting out excess alcohol consumption, improving diet and engaging in regular exercise [41, 42]. Dietary intake of antioxidant supplements has been found efficacious in treating liver diseases [43]. Standard fluid, mineral and vitamin replacement are mandatory in patients hospitalized with liver diseases.

Abstinence from alcohol consumption in patients with alcoholic liver disease is necessary to avoid rapid acceleration of liver disease [44]. Anti-viral medications are available to treat hepatitis liver infections. Other treatment methods involve using steroid-based drugs, anti-tumor necrosis factor, ursodeoxycholic acid and venesection (in hemochromatosis).

Liver transplantation is the only option for those with irreversible liver failure. Most transplants are done for chronic liver diseases leading to cirrhosis, such as chronic hepatitis C, alcoholism, autoimmune hepatitis, and many others. Liver transplant donors are scarce and there are usually long lists of recipients waiting for liver transplant in hospitals.

Diagnosis

Liver disease can be difficult to diagnose in cases where patient show no clinical symptoms. Most patients may have already suffered extensive liver damage before symptoms are observed. However, some of the clinical signs of liver diseases show jaundice, swollen abdomen or tenderness in the area of the liver. Moreover, the diagnosis of liver diseases is made by liver function tests, which are groups of blood tests that can readily show the extent of liver damage [45]. When infection is suspected in the liver, other serological tests can also be carried out. The liver can be physically examined to reveal its size and tenderness. However in some cases, additional imaging is usually required. Ultrasound is the device used to produce an image of the liver. Biopsy is carried out in situations where the cause of liver damage is unknown. In the 21st century they were largely replaced by high-resolution radiographic scans.

Role of Diet in Liver Disease

Diet plays significant roles in liver diseases [46]. They could aid in the progression or in the management of liver diseases thus playing either beneficial or harmful roles. Standardized liver diets are usually designed to necessitate that patients suffering from liver diseases have their nutritional needs met. Many factors are considered in the development of a standardized liver diet due to variations in the different types of liver diseases, nutritional requirements, the stages of the liver disease and other associated medical disorders such as diabetes and cardiovascular disease. Patients with advanced liver diseases are usually recommended a diet providing adequate calories, protein, minerals and vitamins.

Dietary Requirements of Patients Suffering from Liver Disease

Patients with acute liver diseases such as acute viral hepatitis may tolerate food and thus are required to eat normally, as they require more protein and energy. Such patients may benefit from consuming a high protein, high calorie diet. However, suggestions have been made about lipid restrictions in the diet of patients with acute liver diseases such as acute hepatitis and parenchymal liver cells, though this lipid restriction has not shown beneficial role in most acute liver diseases. In fact, they have been suggested to offer advantages to liver disease patients who suffer anorexia by accelerating recovery and decreasing convalescence time [47]. Nutritional supplementations and intravenous fluids are also reserved for patients with anorexia who become malnourished and have difficulty in maintaining sufficient fluid balance. Patients with chronic liver diseases are required to avoid excess calorie consumption particularly carbohydrates as they promote hepatic lipogenesis, increase CO_2 production, liver dysfunction and increase the work of breathing [48]. However, carbohydrates should be sufficient to maintain normal blood glucose levels, and should not exceed insulin reserves and as such patients often do better on multiple small meals with a late bed-time meal, which has been shown to reduce the need for gluconeogenesis, conserve proteins and nitrogen balance after an overnight fast [49].

Fat, in form of polyunsaturated fatty acids with less than 50% long chain triglycerides, should be provided in patients suffering from chronic liver diseases. Fat improves the taste of food and is important in people who suffer from a suppressed appetite due to chronic liver diseases. Without some adequate intake of fat, there would be vitamin deficiency even when vitamin supplements are taken. This type of vitamin deficiency sometimes occurs in people with cholestatic diseases, such as primary biliary cirrhosis. Proteins should not be restricted in patients with chronic liver diseases unless they become protein intolerant due to encephalopathy, though they tolerate vegetable protein better. A high protein diet is important in people with chronic liver diseases as the protein is used to maintain muscles and body tissues such as the liver so as to keep them functioning properly. Moreover, several studies have shown that a daily protein supply of 1.0-1.2 g/kg/day may be sufficient to prevent negative nitrogen balance in cirrhosis [50]. This has to increase by 1.5 g/kg/day in mild stress, and 2.0 g/kg/day in acute exacerbations of hepatitis. Minerals are also important in dietary requirement of patients suffering from chronic liver diseases. Patients with chronic liver diseases are at increased risk for the development of osteoporosis, thus it is important to consume foods rich in calcium and to supplement their diets with calcium. Additionally, zinc supplementation inhibits hepatic inflammation and hepatic fibrosis in patients suffering from chronic liver diseases. However the dietary intake of sodium needs to be restricted as it has been associated with advanced liver diseases. Dietary iron should also be regulated as the body has a limited ability to eliminate excess iron from the body. Excess iron ingestion is usually stored in the liver, predisposing it to toxicity.

Dietary Related Factors Causing Liver Diseases

Obesity is one of the main causes of liver diseases. Obesity is associated with the development of parenchymal liver damage and the formation of gall stones. Occasionally, obese patients develop an inflammation that is histologically similar to alcoholic hepatitis with the formation of Mallory hyaline bodies termed "Non Alcoholic Steatohepatitis NASH." The lesion is not related to the degree of obesity but is occasionally preceded by a short period of weight loss. This is usually a mild slowly progressive lesion, but could progress to cirrhosis.

Vitamin toxicity as a result of vitamin overdose can lead to liver complications. Vitamins must pass through the liver to be metabolized and when taken in excess they have the potential to cause serious health problems. Moreover vitamins are stored in the liver and could reach their storage limits. One of such complication is seen in hypervitaminosis A, which occurs as a result of prolong exposure to high doses of vitamin A in the range of 100,000 U daily in adults. The liver manifestations include hepatomegaly, with hypertrophy of fat storing cells, fibrosis, central vein sclerosis, and cirrhosis. The liver might also undergo changes that lead to vitamin or mineral deficiencies. Low vitamin levels are associated with excessive bleeding, osteoporosis, anemia and night blindness.

Protein energy malnutrition is another diet related cause of liver diseases. Clinical signs of protein-energy malnutrition are frequently seen in cirrhotic patients and may be obvious at all clinical stages of liver diseases and even in clinically stable situations [51]. Protein energy malnutrition is present in 20% of patients with compensated liver diseases and greater than 60% of patients with severe liver insufficiency. However protein energy malnutrition is frequently under diagnosed in clinical practice because water retention increases body weight and thus masks losses of body mass. Protein energy malnutrition is associated with an increased morbidity, mortality and an increased rate of complications such as the persistence of ascites, gastrointestinal bleeding, encephalopathy and increased rate of infections.

Aflatoxins are natural occurring mycotoxins that are derived from the Aspergillus flavus (species of fungi). Aflatoxin-producing members of Aspergillus colonize and contaminate grain before harvest or during storage especially when exposed to a high humid environment or conditions such as drought. The affected grains and legumes include corn, sorghum, groundnut, soybeans, wheat, oat, rice and cotton seed. However, corn remains the most commonly affected grain. Aflatoxins are toxic and amongst the most carcinogenic substances known [52]. They are metabolized by the liver into reactive epoxide intermediate. The epoxide intermediate intercalates into DNA and alkylates the bases through epoxide moiety which can result in the mutations in the p53 gene. High-level aflatoxin exposure produces an acute hepatic necrosis, resulting later in cirrhosis or hepatocellular carcinoma. Aflatoxin levels in food have been found to correlate with the incidence of hepatocellular carcinoma in several areas of Africa and Asia. Moreover hepatocellular carcinoma as a result of chronic aflatoxin exposure has been well documented presenting most often in persons with chronic hepatitis B virus [40]. Aflatoxin probably alters cellular immune response and may increase the carrier rate for hepatitis B.

The aflatoxins known are B_1, B_2, G_1, G_2, M_1 and M_2. Aflatoxin B_1 is the most potent natural occurring chemical liver carcinogen known. Aflatoxins M_1 and M_2 occur in milk unlike the other aflatoxins and they were discovered in the milk of cows fed on moldy grain. Animals do not have high tolerance for aflatoxin exposure as compared to humans who rarely succumb to acute aflatoxicosis [53]. Measures to manage aflatoxin level include minimizing the pre-harvest infection with sound agronomic practices and minimizing post-harvest fungal growth with careful handling and good storage practices. Moreover medical research indicates that a regular diet rich in apiaceous vegetables like carrots, celery, parsley and parsnips reduce the carcinogenic effect of aflatoxin [54].

Role of Antioxidant in Liver Diseases

Several liver diseases are associated with oxidative stress; accordingly antioxidants are believed to serve as therapeutics for the management of various liver diseases. Antioxidant therapy has been suggested to have the possibility of beneficial effects on the liver. Some of these antioxidant therapies include vitamins (A, C, E), some trace minerals (Se, Zn) and certain plant extracts. Their ability to lower oxidative stress plays a significant role in their beneficial effects, though there has been controversy on the beneficial effects of antioxidants in management of liver diseases. A Cochrane database meta-analysis examined 20 randomized clinical trials that used a different antioxidants consisting of selenium, vitamin C, vitamin E and selenium to evaluate their effect on the progression of hepatitis liver disease and liver cirrhosis. They concluded that there was no suitable evidence to support or refute antioxidants in patients with liver diseases, however it was suggested that antioxidants increased the liver enzyme activity [55].

However another study carried out by a group of researchers from the University of Alabama suggested that antioxidants may prevent alcohol liver disease. They introduced an antioxidant to the mitochondria of rats that were given alcohol every day and discovered that the antioxidant was able to counteract the free radicals produced before they were able to damage the mitochondria. Thus this prevented the development of steatosis which would have caused further liver complications [56]. Another study reported that the activities of liver enzymes were significantly increased with the administration of vitamin C in rats [57].

Role of Polyunsaturated Fatty Acids in Liver Diseases

Polyunsaturated fatty acids (PUFAs) are hydrocarbon chains containing more than one double bond. PUFAs can be classified into omega 3 (*n-3*) polyunsaturated fatty acid and omega 6 (*n-6)* polyunsaturated fatty acid according to the position of the double bond at the omega end of the hydrocarbon chain. The omega 3 PUFAs and omega 6 PUFAs are both essential for human health as they regulate a wide variety of biological functions, though they play different roles. Omega-3 PUFAs exert suppressive effects on inflammation while omega 6 PUFAs initiate the inflammatory process. This has attached great importance to the ratio of omega 6 to omega 3 PUFAs in the diet as serious imbalances in favour of omega 6 PUFAs promote the development of several chronic diseases while increased levels of omega 3 PUFAs exert suppressive effects. Moreover, it has been reported that a higher ratio of omega 6 to omega 3 PUFAs in the liver of NAFLD patients may contribute to fatty liver development due to a deranged ability to regulate lipid metabolism in the liver [58].

Polyunsaturated fatty acids occurring in the form of omega 6 PUFAs have been associated with liver complications when excess is consumed in the diet at the expense of omega 3 PUFAs. This is due to the fact that omega 6 PUFAs create a pathological state of proinflammation which is involved in the pathogenesis of NAFLD that represents the hepatic component of most metabolic syndromes. These fatty acids play steatogenic roles and the mechanisms through they promote NAFLD include oxidative stress and increased expression of the proinflammatory cytokines. This has enabled diets high in omega 6 PUFAs to also promote liver cancer. Researchers studied the effect of these fatty acids in development of liver cancer and found out that there was DNA-damaging adducts found in the liver cells of rodents and humans fed on high omega 6 PUFAs. Moreover, omega 6 PUFAs have been related to liver damage in asymptomatic patients with HIV infections [59].

The omega-3 PUFAs however, suppress the inflammatory pumps and have been found more suitable in patients with liver diseases. Animal studies have shown that omega 3 polyunsaturated fatty acid enriched diets caused the development of steatohepatitis and reduced hepatic triglyceride content [60]. The benefit is thought to be as a result of the modulation of lipid processing by omega-3 fatty acid in acting as ligands of the peroxisome proliferator-activated receptor α (PPARα) and reducing hepatic inflammation, as well as combating oxidative stress [61]. Another study also reported that consumption of omega 3 rich fish oil was beneficial in reducing NAFLD in patients [62]. They observed that the omega-3 PUFAs decrease plasma non esterified fatty acid concentration, lipogenesis and adipocyte fat storage.

Role of Branched Amino Acid in Liver Diseases

Branched chain amino acids (BCAAs) comprise of amino acids with a branched or side chain. Branched chain amino acids have been found useful in muscles generation and they also play an important role in signaling chemicals in the brain. However, BCAAs have now been found to play a prominent role in the management of liver diseases [63]. Malnutrition is a recurrent feature in chronic liver diseases because such liver disease patients lack amino acids, which serve as the building block of proteins. Specifically, there has been reported decrease in serum levels of branched chain amino acids in patients with liver Cirrhosis, which contributes to the prognosis of the disease [64]. Moreover, the ongoing energy and protein catabolism in such patients with chronic liver diseases is responsible for the decreases in amino acids. The increase in muscle protein degradation accompanied by the impairment of liver function produces an imbalance in plasma amino acid pattern which results in an elevation of aromatic amino acids and a reduction of branched amino acids. It is suggested that this imbalance plays a key role in the pathophysiology of hepatic encephalopathy and involves in protein intolerance in such patients. This contributes to the necessity of an additional nutritional requirement in patients with chronic liver diseases. The supplementation of diet with BCAAs has proven to be very useful. BCAAs have been found to increase protein synthesis in the liver of patients suffering from chronic liver diseases. Thus effectively managing the disease and improving the quality of life of the patient.

There has been conflicting data supporting the beneficial role of BCAAs in managing patient with liver diseases, however there are more evidences against this notion. BCAAs have been found very useful in patients suffering from chronic liver diseases. a study on 48 patients was carried out [65]. Twenty four patients had chronic hepatic encephalopathy and were administered BCAAs and 24 patients serving as controls were used in the study. There was significant improvement and recovery from chronic hepatic encephalopathy in patients who received BCAA administration compared to the control group. There was also a significant decrease and increase in ammonia and albumin respectively. Another study carried out [66] demonstrated that branched chain amino acid enriched snacks improved the liver functioning of patients with liver cirrhosis who had undergone radiofrequency ablation for hepatocellular carcinoma. BCAAs have also been found to improve glucose metabolism in rats with liver cirrhosis [67]. It was also reported that BCAA supplemented in the diet of rats caused a delay in progression of chronic liver diseases by attenuating hepatic apoptosis in rats induced with carbon tetrachloride to facilitate a liver damage [68].

COMMON HEPATOPROTECTIVE FOODS OR FRUITS

Some of the plants commonly consumed as food are rich in phytochemicals and nutrient that boost the hepatoprotective ability of such plants. Different parts of these plants such as the fruit, seed, stem or root may be consumed as a food. Thus the consumption of these food plants rich in the necessary phytochemicals and nutrients offers additional medicinal advantage apart from a normal consumption as foods due to taste, tolerability and ability to supply the needed energy for the body.

Garlic has been found to possess important dietary and medicinal role for centuries. Most of its therapeutic properties are due to the specific oil and water soluble organosulfur compounds present. There are a variety of antioxidants in garlic which protects against diseases caused by oxidative damages. The antioxidant phytochemicals include terpenoids, flavnoids and phenols [69]. Garlic extract provides hepatoprotection by lowering the alanine transaminase (ALT), alkaline phosphatase (ALP), and albumin level. They also inhibit lipid peroxidation in the liver. In combination with silymarin, a well-known hepatoprotectant and clove oil, garlic extract shows hepatoprotective activity in N-nitrosodiethylamine with CCl_4 and lead-induced hepatotoxicity, respectively [70]. Pharmacokinetics of specific components of garlic extract has not been studied well in detail. Overall, garlic provides a good level of hepatoprotection in preclinical animal models.

Red chili is a member of genus Capsicum and family Solanaceae. The fruit is mainly used as a spice and food vegetable in most countries. However, they have found considerable use in medicine. They possess a wide array of phytochemicals with well known antioxidant properties. Some of the antioxidative phytochemicals contained include flavanoids, querctin, luteolin, carotenoids and capsaicnoids. The main active constituent of chili is capsaicin (8-methyl-N-vanilyl-6-nonenamide) along with other chemical constituents. A study has shown that capsaicin acts as proapototic factor for cancerous liver cells and suggested that capsaicin may be beneficial in therapeutic intervention of hepatoma [71].

Apple, referred to as Pyrus malus (botanical name), is the most widely used fruit across the world. Apple fruit tree is perennial and member of family Rosaceae. The healthy benefits of apples are numerous as they support the human health when eaten raw or cooked. Apple extracts have been studied and they prove great antioxidant effects [72]. Apple polyphenol treatment reduces ALT and AST level in CCl_4-induced hepatotoxicity. A study reported that apple polyphenol-treated mice also show reduced malondialdehyde, reduced level of GSH, increased level of superoxide dismutase, and reduced lipid peroxidation [73].

Carrot, also known as Daucus carota, is a biennial herb of family Apiaceae. Edible part of carrot is root. Carrots were first used for medical purposes and gradually used as food. Carrots contain carotenoids, anthocyanin, flavanoids, polyphenols and polyacetylenes [74]. It is also a rich source of dietary fiber, minerals (magnesium, manganese, molybydenum, phosphorus, and potassium), vitamins (vit A, vit b, vit C, vit E and vit K). It has been widely used as remedy of jaundice in Europe. Carrot extracts show good hepatoprotective activity using CCl_4-induced liver injury in Wistar rats [75]. Administration of carrot extract to experimental rats also resulted in decreased bilirubin and urea levels.

Sweet corn referred to as Zea mays var. saccharata, also known as Indian corn or sugar corn is a variety of maize. Sweet corn seed is widely used in many vegetarian dishes across the globe. It contains ferulic acid than other fruits or vegetables. Ferulic acid is an important antioxidant that prevents oxidative damage in several diseases [76]. They may also have some implications in hepatoprotective activity of sweet corn. Corn peptides possess hepatoprotective activity in vivo using internal liver injury mice model [77]. Moreover, the hepatoprotective activity of corn peptide was found significant at a dosage of 600 mg/kg bodyweight, and its hepatoprotective activity is found close to well-known hepatoprotective herb silymarin.

Soybean, also referred to as *Glycine max* has high antioxidant property. It is rich in health promoting phytochemicals and contains saponins, isoflavones, phytic acid, lignans, phytosterols and phenolic acid. The isoflavones compounds present in soybean are responsible for its high antioxidative activity [78]. Interestingly, in a cohort-based study in Japan, it has been found that soy consumption may reduce the risk of hepatitis C virus [79].

Coffee powder is roasted seed of coffee beans. Coffee is rich in antioxidants. In fact, it has showed more antioxidant activity than green tea. Phenolics and melanoidins are main bioactive constituents of coffee brew [80]. Coffee consumption has shown beneficial effect in different kinds of liver diseases like cirrhosis, hepatitis B and hepatitis C virus infection. It was showed that coffee extract and its constituents had inhibitory effect on hepatitis B virus replication in HepG2.2.25 cells as well as in duck hepatitis B virus replication model [81]. An inverse correlation has also been established between increased coffee consumption and a decrease risk of cirrhosis.

Turmeric or Curcuma longa is a widely used spice in India and other neighboring countries. It has a peppery, warm and bitter flavor. It belongs to the ginger family. It is best known as one of the ingredients used to make "curry" a food condiment. Tumeric has been used in traditional medicine for the treatment of various ailments. The main bioactive compound isolated from turmeric is a yellow color pigment known as curcumin [82]. Curcumin exhibits a wide range of pharmacological activities including anti-inflammatory, antitumor, antioxidative, and free radical scavenging activity. Tumeric also increase detoxification system in the liver. In vitro as well as in vivo animal studies have indicated the hepatoprotective effect of curcumin in case of different hepatotoxic stresses caused due to carbon tetrachloride (CCl_4), paracetamol, galactosamine, pentobarbital and 1-chloro-2,4-dinitrobenzene. It also exhibits chemopreventive effect against hepatocarcinogenesis. It was showed that curcumin possesses antiproliferative, antiinvasive, and proapoptotic activity in various hepatocellular carcinoma (HCC)-derived cell lines [83].

Coriander with the botanical name of Coriandrum sativum is one of the most important herbs used as a spice and flavoring agent. Coriander fruit is mostly present in all kinds of mixed spices used in India and other Asian countries. The dry seeds and the fresh leaves are the part most traditionally used in cooking. Coriander seeds promote the hepatic antioxidant system [84]. Hepatoprotective activity of essential oil of coriander has been studied in CCl_4-induced hepatotoxicity in rat. It was showed that administration of coriander oil had significant free radical scavenging activity and improved production of different antioxidative enzymes [85].

Grape is a perennial vine, member of genus Vitis. Vitis vinifera (grape) fruit is used as a food and for making wine, jam, jellies, juice, vinegar and grape seed extract. Resveratrol is the main bioactive constituent of grape. It is a potent anti-inflammatory and antioxidant molecule. Resveratrol treatment to hepatoma-bearing mice have shown dramatic reduction in tumor volume and increased survival of experimental rat [86]. In vitro studies have shown that resveratrol inhibits proliferation and also acts as proapoptotic agent when administered to different hepatoma cell lines [87]. Grape also contains anthocyanins, the main polyphenolics in purple grapes. Anthocyanin confers some hepatoprotective effect as well as they have even been suggested as nutritional therapy for nonalcoholic fatty liver diseases.

Pomegranate or Punica granatum is a deciduous shrub of genus Punica and family Lythraceae. The most abundant phytochemicals in pomegranate juice are polyphenols and hydrolysable tannins. Anthocyanins are also present in the juice. The crude pomegranate juice exhibits a strong antioxidative and antiproliferative property in comparison to the purified polyphenol components of pomegranate juice. Moreover, pomegranate juice consumption reduces oxidative stress [88]. The pomegranate peel extract also possesses a strong hepatoprotective activity. The peel extract treatment reduces serum AST, ALT, and lactate dehydrogenase level significantly [89].

Green tea is derived from the leaves of Camellia sinensis, a member of family Theaceae. It has been a widely used drink worldwide as far back as 5000 years ago. Green tea is rich in phytochemicals such as polyphenols, flavanols and caffeine [90]. They are also rich in catechins. Catechins are very powerful antioxidants [91]. Green tea provides hepatoprotection against variety of hepatotoxic agents like naphthoquinone and alcohol. Generally green tea reduces the risk of developing liver cancer.

Conclusion

Diet thus plays a very important role in liver diseases as it has been found both beneficial and harmful in liver diseases. Thus diet related factors should be monitored closely in etiology of liver diseases as they contribute significantly towards hepatoprotective effects or liver damaging effects.

References

[1] Cotran R, Kumar S, Fausto N, Nelso F, Robbins SL, Abbas AK. Robbins and Cotran pathologic basis of disease (7th ed.). St. Louis, MO: Elsevier Saunders; 2005. p. 878.

[2] Maton A, Jean H, Charles W, Susan J, Maryanna W, David L, et al. Human Biology and Health. Englewood Cliffs, New Jersey, USA: Prentice Hall; 1993.

[3] Häussinger D. Liver Regeneration. Berlin: De Gruyter; 2011. p. 1.

[4] Shyamal S, Latha P, Suja D, Shine V, Anuja G, Sini S, et al. Hepatoprotective effect of three herbal extracts on aflatoxin B1 intoxicated rat liver. *Singerpore Med. J.* 2010; 51(4): 326.

[5] Krishna K, Hilman J. Kundalini – the evolutionary energy in man. London: Stuart and Watkins; 1970. p. 77.

[6] Uthandi A, Ramasamy K. Hepatoprotective activity of sesame meal on high fat fed rats. *Intern J. Pharma Sci. Res*. 2011; 2(12): 205-211.

[7] Zwicky C, Gerber S, Gasparini D, Forestier F, Hohlfeld P, Tissot J, Schneider P. Preparation and Analysis of Fetal liver extracts. *Bone Marrow Transpl. J.* 2000; 26(6):667-671.

[8] Zakim D, Boyer, Thomas D. Hepatology: A Textbook of Liver Disease (4th ed.). Philadelphia: Saunders; 2002.

[9] McGorrin RJ. Food analysis techniques: Introduction. In: Encyclopedia of Analytical Chemistry. John Wiley and Sons, Ltd.; 2006. DOI:10. 1002/9780470027318.a1001.

[10] Ros K. Energy and fuel. In: Ross KA, Lakin E (eds). Science knowledge and the Environment. London: David Fulton Publishers; 2000.

[11] Mahmoed MY, Rezq AA. Hepatoprotective effect of Avocado fruits against Carbon Tetrachloride- induced liver damage in male rats. *World Appl. Sci. J.* 2013; 21(10):1445-1452.

[12] Bellows L, Moore R. Fat soluble vitamins: A, D, E and K. Colarado State University Extension; 2012.

[13] Xu K, Morgan K, Todd G, Elston T, Gomez S. A whole body model for glycogen regulation reveals a critical role for substrate cycling in maintaining blood glucose homeostatasis. *PLoS Comput. Biol*. 2011; 7(12):e1002272.

[14] Schneewind JH, Fuller JB, Cole WH. The importance of protein metabolism and liver function in Gaeratic surgical patients. *Off. J. Am. Geriat Soc.* 1957; 5(1):1-7.

[15] Nguyen P, Leray V, Diez M, Serisier S, Bloc J, Siliart B, et al. Liver lipid metabolism. *J. Anim. Physiol. Anim. Nutr*. 2008; 92(3):272-283.

[16] Steven G. Chronic Liver Disease. *J. Gener. Intern. Med*. 2000; 15(2):142.

[17] Matteoni C, Younossi Z, Gramlich T. NON-alcoholic fatty liver disease: a spectrum of clinical and pathological severity. *Gastroentorol.* 1999; 116:1413-9.

[18] Beckingham IJ. ABC of diseases of liver, pancreas and biliary system: investigation of liver and biliary disease. *BMJ*. 2001; 322(7277):33-6.

[19] Wong C, Goh K. Chronic hepatitis B infection and liver cancer. *Biomed. Imaging Interv*. 2006; 2(3):7.

[20] de Oliveira Andrade LJ, D'Oliveira A, Melo RC, De Souza EC, Costa Silva CA, Parana R. Association between Hepatitis C and hepatocellular carcinoma. *J. Glob. Infect Dis*. 2009; 1(1):33-37.

[21] Civan J, Hann H. Hepatitis C virus mediated hepatocellular carcinoma: A focused review for a time of changing therapeutic options. *North Am. J. Med. Sci.* 2014; 7(1):8-16.

[22] Vernon G, Baranova A, Younossi Z. Systematic review: the epidemiology and natural history of non-alcoholic fatty liver disease and non-alcoholic steatohepatitis in adults. *Aliment Pharmacol. Ther*. 2011; 34:274-285.

[23] Lazo M, Clark J. The epidemiology of non-alcoholic fatty liver disease: a global perspective. *Semin. Liver Dis*. 2008; 28:339-350.

[24] Bellentani S, Scagilioni F, Marino M, Bedgoni G. Epidiemology of non-alcoholic fatty liver disease. *Dig. Dis*. 2011; 28(1):1555-61.

[25] Stevenson M, Lloyd-Jones M, Morgan M, Wrong R. Non-invasive diagnostic assessment tools for the detection of liver fibrosis in patients with suspected alcohol

related liver disease. A systematic review and economic evaluation. *Health Technol. Assess.* 2012; 16(4):1-174.

[26] Singal A, Anand B. Recent trends in the epidemiology of alcoholic liver disease. *Clin. Liver Dis.* 2013; 2:53-56.

[27] Lok A, Heathcote E, Hoofnagle J. Management of hepatitis B: 2000 Summary of a workshop. *Gastroenterol.* 2001; 120:1828-1853.

[28] Daniel L. Global burden of hepatitis C. *Liver international* 2009; 29:74-81.

[29] Sharma A, Chakraborti K, Handa S. Anti-hepatotoxic activity of some Indian herbal formulations as compared to silymarin. *Fitoterapia* 1991; 62:229-235.

[30] Alan P, Christos P, Junji F, Laura G. The incidence and epidemiology of hepatocellular carcinoma: a global regional perspective. *Oncol.* 2010; 15(4):513.

[31] Poon D, Anderson B, Chen L. Management of hepatocellular carcinoma in Asia: Consensus statement from the Asian Oncology summit. *Lancet Oncol.* 2009; 10:11111118.

[32] Cusi K. Role of insulin resistance and lipotoxicity in non-alcoholic steatohepatitis. *Clin. Liver Dis.* 2009; 13:545-563.

[33] Reddy J, Rao M. Lipid metabolism and liver inflammation. Fatty liver disease and fatty acid oxidation. *Am. J. Physiol. Gastrointest. Liver Physiol.* 2006; 290 (5):52-8.

[34] Eduardo R, Leonor R, Eunate G, Eva M, Mar G. Lipotoxicity, fatty acid uncoupling and mitochondria carrier function. *Biochem. Biophys. Bioenergetics.* 2010; 1797(7):800-806.

[35] Cunningham C, Van Horn C. Energy availability and alcohol-related liver pathology. *Alcohol Res. Health.* 2003; 27:b291–9.

[36] Wu D, Cederbaum A. Alcohol, oxidative stress, and free radical damage. *Alcohol Res. Health.* 2003; 27:277–84.

[37] Hoek J, Pastorino J. Cellular signaling mechanisms in alcohol-induced liver damage. *Semin. Liver Dis.* 2004; 24:257–72.

[38] Vergani D, Miel G. Mechanism of autoimmune hepatitis. *Pediatr Transplantr.* 204; 8(6):589-93.

[39] Haber P, Warner R, Seth D, Gorell M, McCaughan G. Pathogenesis and management of alcoholic hepatitis. *Journal of Gastrointestinal Hepatol.* 2003; 18(12):1332-44.

[40] Yan L, Felicia W. Global burden of Aflatoxin induced hepatocellular carcinoma: A risk assessment. *Environ. Health Project.* 2010; 118(6):818-824.

[41] Hickman IJ, Jonsson JR, Prins JB. Modest weight loss and physical activity in overweight patients with chronic liver disease results in sustained improvements in alanine aminotransferase, fasting insulin, and quality of life. *Gut* 2004; 53(3):413–9.

[42] Nobili V, Manco M, Devito R. Lifestyle intervention and antioxidant therapy in children with nonalcoholic fatty liver disease: a randomized, controlled trial. *Hepatol.* 2008; 48(1):119-28.

[43] Bjelakovic G, Gluud L, Nikolova D, Bjelakovic M, Nagorni A, Gluud C. Antioxidant supplement for liver diseases. *Cochrane Datab. Syst. Rev.* 2011; Issue 3, Article No.: CD007749. DOI: 10.1002/14651858. CD007749.pub2.

[44] Nimela O. Biomarkers in alcoholism. *Clin Chim Acta.* 2007; 377:39-49.

[45] Shivaraj G, Prakash B, Vinayak H, Avinash A, Sonal N, Shruth K. A review on laboratory liver function test. *Pan. Afr. Med.* 2009; 3:17.

[46] Nicole J, Lydia A, Marco M, Michelle M. Phenotyping the effect of diet on non – alcoholic fatty liver disease. *J. Hepatol.* 2012; 57(6):1370-1373.

[47] Crews RH, Faloon WW. The fallacy of a low fat diet in liver disease. *JAMA*. 1962; 181(9):754-759.

[48] Sevastianova K, Santos A, Kotronen A, Hakkarainen A, Makkonen J, Silander K, et al. Effect of short term carbohydrate over feeding and long term weight loss on liver fat in overweight humans. *Am. J. Clin. Nutr.* 2012; 96(4):724-34.

[49] Bertelsen J, Christiansen C, Thomsen C, Poulsen PL, Vestergaard S, Steinov A. Effect of meal frequency on blood glucose, insulin and free fatty acids in NIDDM subjects. *Eur. J. Clin. Nutr.* 1993; 16(1):4-7.

[50] Sareh E, Hossein P, Reza M. Malnutrition in liver cirrhosis: the influence of protein and sodium. *Middle East J. Dig. Dis*. 2013; 5(2):65-75.

[51] Huisman EJ. Protein energy malnutrition predicts complications in liver cirrhosis. *Eur. J. Gastroenterol. Hepatol*. 2011; 23(11):982-9.

[52] Hudler G. Magical mushrooms, mischievious molds: The remarkable story of the Fungus kingdom and its impact on Human affairs. Princeton University Press; 1998.

[53] Williams J, Philips T, Jolly P, Stiles J, Jolly C, Aggarwal D. Human aflatoxicosis in developing countries: A review of toxicology, exposure, potential health consequences and interventions. *Am. J. Clin. Nutr.* 2004; 80(5):1106-22.

[54] Peterson S, Lampe JW, Bammler TK, Gross-Steinmeyer K, Eaton DL. Apiaceous vegetable constituents inhibit human cytochrome P-450 1A2 (hCYP1A2) activity and hCYP1A2- mediated mutagenicity of aflatoxin B1. *Fd. Chem. Toxicol.* 2006; 44(9):1474-84.

[55] Bjelacovik G, Gluud L, Nicolova D, Bjelacovik M, Nargoni A, Gluud C. Antioxidant supplement for liver disease. *Cochrane Datab. Syst. Rev.* 2011; Issue 3. Art. No.: CD007749. DOI: 10.1002/14651858. CD007749.pub2.

[56] Balu K, Anup S, Michelle J, Gloria A, Jung C, Yaozu Y. The mitochondria targerted Ubiquinone Mito-Q decreases ethanol dependent macro amd micro hepatosteatosis. *Hepatol.* 2011; 54(1):153-63.

[57] Karakilsic A. Effect of Vitamin C on liver enzyme and biochemical parameters in rats anesthetized with halothane. *Gen. Physol. Biophys.* 2005; 24(1):47-55.

[58] Patterson E, Wall R, Filtzgerald G, Ross R, Stanton C. Health implications of high dietary omega-6 polyunsaturated fatty acid. *J. Nutr. Metab.* 2012; 2:539426.

[59] Oosthuizen W, Van G, Kruger A, Vorster H. Polyunsaturated fatty acid intake is adversely related to liver function in HIV- infected subjects: the THUSA Study. *Am. J. Clin. Nutr.* 2006; 83(5):1193-8.

[60] Mummadi RR, Kasturi KS, Chennareddygari S. Effect of bariatric surgery on nonalcoholic fatty liver disease: systematic review and meta-analysis. *Clin. Gastroenterol. Hepatol*. 2008; 6(12):1396-402.

[61] Reddy J, Rao M. Lipid metabolism and liver inflammation. Fatty liver disease and fatty acid oxidation. *Am. J. Physiol. Gastrointest. Liver Physiol*. 2006; 290(5):52-8.

[62] Minno M, Rusollilo A, Lupoli R, Ambrosino P, Minno A, Tarantino G. Omega-3 fatty acid for the treatment of non alcoholic fatty liver disease. *World J. Gastroenterol*. 2012; 18(41):5839-5847.

[63] Knanna S, Gopalan S. Role of Branched Chain Amino acids in liver disease The evidence for and against. *Curr. Opin. Clin. Nutr. Metab. Care.* 2007; 10(3):297-303.

[64] Kazuto T, Yukihiro S. Branched chain amino acids in liver diseases. *World J. Gastroenterol.* 2013; 19(43):7620-7629.

[65] Somro A, Devrajani B, Ghori H, Lohana H, Quereshi A(2008). Role of brached chain amino acid in the management of hepatic encephalopathy. *World Journal of Medical Sciences*. 3(2):60-64.

[66] Morihara D, Iwata K, Hanano T, Kunimoto H, Kuno S. Late-evening snack with branched-chain amino acids improves liver function after radiofrequency ablation for hepatocellular carcinoma. *Hepatol. Res.* 2012; 18(33):4486-4490.

[67] Nishitani S, Takehana K, Fujitani S, Sonaka I. Branched Chain amino acid improve glucose metabolism in rats with liver cirrhosis. *Am. J. Physiol. Gastrointest Liver Physiol.* 2005; 288(6):G1292-300.

[68] Masashi K, Hiroyo K, Hiroaki K, Shunsuke I, Aki O, Yukiko K. Suplementation with branched chain amino acid attenuates hepatic apoptosis in rats with chronic liver disease. *Nutr. Res.* 2012; 32(7):522-9.

[69] Elena A, Alessandra D, Maria S, Olindo T, Eugenia V, Simona V, et al. Phytochemical content in Italian garlic bulb varieties. *J. Food Res.* 2014; 3:4.

[70] Ajai G, Adeniyi T, Babayemi D. Hepatoprotective and some haematological aspects of Allium sativum and vitamin C in lead-exposed Wistar rats. *Intern J. Med. Med. Sci.* 2009; 1:64–67.

[71] Lee Y, Kang Y, Lee J, Nicolova S, Kim J. Involvement of NADPH oxidase mediated generation of reactive oxygen species in the apoptotic cell death by capsaicin in HepG2 human hepatoma cells. *Free Rad. Res.* 2004; 38:405–412.

[72] Marian V, Chang Y, Rui H. Nutrition: Antioxidant activity of fresh apples. *Nature* 2000; 405(22):903-904.

[73] Yang J, Li Y, Wang F, Wu C (2010). Hepatoprotective effect of apple polyphenols on CCL4 induced acute liver damage in mice. *J. Agric. Food Chem.* 2010; 10: 6525–6531.

[74] Dias J. Nutritional and health benefit of carrot and their seed extracts. *Food Nutr. Sci.* 2014; 5:2147-2156.

[75] Bishayee A, Sarkar A, Chatterjee M. Hepatoprotective activity of carrot (Daucus carota L.) against carbon tetrachloride intoxication in mouse liver. *J. Ethnopharmacol.* 1995; 47:69–74.

[76] Dewanto V, Wu X, Hai R. Processed Sweet Corn has higher antioxidant activity. *J. Agric. Food Chem.* 2002; 50(17):4959-4964.

[77] Guo G, Sun J, He H. Antihepatotoxic effect of corn peptides against Bacillus Calmette–Guerin/lipopolysaccharide-induced liver injury in mice. *Food Chem. Technol.* 2009; 47:2431–2435.

[78] Chao X. Health effects of Soy Protein and Isoflavones in Humans. *J. Nutr.* 2008; 138(6):1244S-9S.

[79] Sharp GB, Lagarde F, Mizuno T, Sauvaget C, Fukuhara T, Allen N, et al. Relationship of hepatocellular carcinoma to soya food consumption: a cohort-based, case–control study in Japan. *Intern J. Cancer.* 2005; 10:290–295.

[80] Coelhot C, Ribeirot M, Cruzt A, Dominguess R, Coimbras M, Bunzel M, et al. Nature of phenolic compounds in coffee melanoidins. *J. Agric. Food Chem.* 2014; 62(31):7843-7853.

[81] Wang G, Shi L, Ren Y. Anti-hepatitis B virus activity of chlorogenic acid, quinic acid and caffeic acid in vivo and in vitro. *Antiv Res.* 2009; 83:186–190.

[82] Monika N and Shaveta S (2013). Role of curcumin in systemic and oral health: An overview. *Journal of Natural Science Biology and Medicine.* 4 (1): 3-7.

[83] Bae MK, Kim SH, Jeong JW. Curcumin inhibits hypoxia induced angiogenesis by down regulation of HIF-1. *Oncol. Rep.* 2006; 15:1557–1562.

[84] Naveen S, Farhath K. Antioxidant potential of Coriander seed extract and its amelioration of liver antioxidant enzymes by CCL_4 induced toxicity in rats. *Intern J. Pharmaceut Biol. Arch.* 2010; 1(4):393-98.

[85] Samojlik I, Lakic N, Mimica-Dukic N, Dakovic-savicer K, Bozin B. Antioxidant and hepatoprotective potential of essential oils of coriander (Coriandrum sativum L.) and caraway (Carum carvi L.) (Apiaceae). *J. Agric. Food Chem.* 2010; 15:8848–8853.

[86] Carbo N, Costelli P, Baccino F. Resveratrol, a natural product present in wine, decreases tumor growth in a rat tumor model. *Biophys. Biochem. Res. Commun.* 1999; 254:739–743.

[87] Bhardwaj A, Sethi G, Vadhan-Raj S, Bueso-Ramos C, Takada Y, Gaur U. Resveratol inhibits proliferation, induces apotosis and overcomes chemoresistance through down regulation of STAT-3 and nuclear factor-kappaB- regulated antiapoptotic and cell survival gene products in human multiple myeloma cells. *Blood J.* 2007; 109(6):2293-302.

[88] Aviram M, Dornfeld L, Rosenblat M, Volkova N, Kaplan M, Coleman R, et al. Pomegranate juice consumption reduces oxidative stress, atherogenic modifications to LDL, and platelet aggregation: studies in humans and in atherosclerotic apolipoprotein E – deficient mice. *Am. J. Clin. Nutr.* 2000; 71(5):1062-76.

[89] Toklu HZ, Dumlu MU, Sehirili O. Pomegranate peel extract prevents liver fibrosis in biliary obstructed rats. *J Pharm and Pharmacol.* 2007; 59:1287–1295.

[90] Olosunde O, Abu-Saeed K, Abu-Saheed M. Phytochemical Screenind and Antimicrobial properties of common brand of black tea (Camellia sinensis) marketed in *Nigerian Environ. Adv. Pharmaceut. Bull.* 2012; 2(2):259-263.

[91] Luper S. A review of plants used in the treatment of liver disease: part two. *Altern Med. Rev.* 1999; 4:178-188.

In: Diets and Diseases: Causes and Prevention
Editor: Wenbiao Wu
ISBN: 978-1-63484-580-9

Chapter 7

DIETS AND BONE DISEASES

Asif Ahmad* and Muhammad Kaleem†
Department of Food Technology,
PMAS-Arid Agriculture University Rawalpindi, Rawalpindi, Pakistan

ABSTRACT

Nutrition related bone problems are very common in all nations across the globe. Over and under intake of certain nutrients is considered the major cause for these problems. Sometimes such problems may arise as a result of internal metabolites. This chapter will discuss the theories related to bone problems keeping in view the hypo and hyper conditions of nutrients in relation to bone related problems such as osteoporosis, osteomalacias, parathyroidism, Paget's disease, fibrous dysplasia and many more. Role of micro and macro minerals in relation to bone disease will also be the topic of discussion. Glimpses from previous research will be presented to gather the evidences that these problems can be well managed through the diet. Diet interaction with other factors such as genetic, medical, pharmacological and modern lifestyle will be viewed in relation to bone health. New techniques for evaluation of bone abnormalities will also be under discussion. Demographic data on bone disease will suggest who is more likely at risk. Finally, scientific strategies will be framed that will suggest some prophylactic measures intended to control the bone diseases through diets.

Keywords: bone disease, osteomalacia, osteoporosis, diet

INTRODUCTION

Bone health of an organism depends upon the achievement of peak bone mass during the development and then the subsequent loss of bone mass i.e., resorption of bone. There are two types of factors that affect the achievement of peak bone mass, firstly factors that cannot be

* Corresponding Author Address: Department of Food Technology, PMAS-Arid Agriculture University Rawalpindi Pakistan, E-mail address: asifahamd@uaar.edu.pk.
† E-mail address: kaleem.ft@gmail.com.

changed like genetics, environment and age etc., and secondly factors that can be changed or modified like diet, smoking habits, alcohol consumption and exercise etc. Among these modifiable factors the most important one is diet, which affects the achievement of peak bone mass and also affects the subsequent bone loss due to aging. Consumption of diet that is deficient in the calcium results in less peak bone mass achievement during development, and in the later life calcium deficient diet increases resorption of bone mass to maintain the level of calcium in the plasma. Calcium is an important constituent for maintaining the healthy bone, there are several other dietary factors which positively or negatively affect the absorption of calcium from diets for example people who are deficient in vitamin D are unable to absorb calcium from the food so they are at greater risk for fracture even though they are consuming a diet which contains appreciable amount of calcium. Another factor which affects the bone is obesity, which is caused by diets and it can also be prevented by changing dietary habits.

Deficiency of dietary calcium is a major cause of osteoporosis that is defined as less quantity of mineralized bone. In comparison to osteoporosis, osteomalacia is caused by the deficiency of vitamin D and it can be defined as defected bone mineralization. Strength of bone is affected by osteomalacia as well as osteoporosis which increase the chances of bone fractures [1]. Bone mass of the organism depends upon the achieved peak bone mass during the growth and development, and on the loss of bone mass later in the life due to aging. So osteoporosis can be prevented by achieving maximum peak bone mass during growth and by reducing bone mass loss in subsequent life which can be achieved by consuming diets rich in calcium [2].

Due to industrialization and change in life style a large proportion of population is not sufficiently exposed to sun light so vitamin D deficiency is increasing in the population. Vitamin D deficiency causes rickets in children and osteomalacia and osteopenia in adults. These diseases can be prevented by consuming a diet which is rich in vitamin D or food products that are fortified with vitamin D. By consuming diet containing appreciable quantity of vitamin D or food product fortified with it, rickets and osteomalcia can be prevented. Osteomalcia and hypocalcemia in CYP27B1 mice were prevented by consuming a diet rich in vitamin D [3]. This study shows the importance of diet for prevention of bone diseases.

Hemostasis of bone is regulated by osteoblast and osteoclasts. Reduction of bone is induced by aging which decreases the formation of bone by osteoblast and increases bone resorption by osteoclast. A major health problem is osteoporosis that results in decreases in bone mass. Osteoporosis is expressed by fractures of femur bone and its incidence increases with increasing age of population [4]. Malnutrition is often observed in patients suffering from fractures [5]. Macro and micro nutrient deficiency is strongly associated with hip fractures pathogenesis and consequences of osteoporosis in aged people. A large number of evidence indicated that bone loss can be prevented by nutritional factors [6]. The effect of diets on bone mineral content and bone area was investigated in 10 yrs old Danish children which showed that BMC and bone area (BA) are positively related with energy intake and different nutrients which include dietary proteins but it was negatively associated with intake of sodium and phosphorus [7].

Carbohydrates are important parts of diets. Among carbohydrates sugars are consumed largely as parts of soft drinks and other beverages. To check the effect of sugar on bone a study was conducted in which mice were fed with fructose rich or glucose rich diets. High fructose fed group showed greater bone volume of distal femur, decreased bone surface and greater thickness of trabeculae. Similarly the flexture load of tibia was found higher in the fructose rich diet. These results showed that a fructose rich diet makes the bone stronger as compared to a diet rich in glucose [8].

CAUSES OF BONE DISEASES

There are two chief sources of vitamin D_3, animal source and internal body synthesis of vitamin D_3. Vegetarian people consume only foods that come from the plant source so for them the source of vitamin D_3 is only internal body synthesis of vitamin D_3. In the certain parts of the world there is not sufficient sun shine for sufficient synthesis of vitamin D_3 or there is a problem for dark skin people because melanin pigment in the skin affects penetration of UV light which converts 7 dehydrocholesterol to cholecalciferol (Vitamin D_3) which is further metabolized in the liver. So more exposure to sun is required for dark skin people for sufficient conversion of 7 dehydrocholesterol to calciferol to maintain the normal level of viamin D in the plasma or they are required to eat foods enriched with vitamin D. Seeking vitamin D_3 importance for bone health, a study was conducted, which analyzed the bone mineral density (BMD) of vegetarian people with non-vegan population. It was concluded that BMD was found to be lower in vegetarian as compared to their counter population [9]. This highlights the importance of a diet for bone health. People who consume vegetarian diets are often deficient from nutrients like calcium, vitamin D and vitamin B_{12} [10, 11]. Vitamin B_{12} deficiency along with folate affects homocysteine (HCY) metabolism and hyperhomocysteine and results in increased bone turn over markers [12] that increase the risk of fractures. People consuming vegetarian diets especially elders women are at higher risk of osteoporosis as compared to non-vegetarian people [13].

Obesity is a global health problem that affects more than 300 million people annually. Obesity is a major risk factor for bone fractures especially osteoporosis and increases the chances of bone fractures [14, 15]. These adverse effects of obesity are attributed by an increase in oxidative stress and inflammation. Epidemiological studies had shown that obesity induced by consumption of high fat diets, or deficiency of estrogen due to menopause and glucocorticoid therapy was inversely related to bone mass [16]. Similarly another study showed that obesity was associated with fragility of bone [17, 18]. These detrimental effects of bone induced from diets can be prevented by consumption of a diet which is rich in vitamin D and calcium as evidenced by obese mice experiments [19]. Similarly, another study showed the consumption of vegetables and fruits helps to prevent obesity as well as osteoporosis [20].

Glucocorticoid therapy is a cause of secondary osteoporosis. Long term glucocorticoid therapy results in 30-50% bone fractures. Glucocorticoid induced osteoporosis results in bi phasic loss of mineral density, 6-12 percent during 1st year and 3 percent per annum thereafter [21]. Glucocorticoid therapy induced osteoporosis can be linked to obesity because higher secretion of glucocorticoid is associated with obesity which in turn is inversely related to bone mass as described above [22]. Deficiency of folic acid during pregnancy, from 1st week of conception till third month of gestation is responsible for neural tube defects. A study was conducted, which showed that deficiency of folic acid decreased level of TGF-B and IGF

[23]. Deficiency of folic acid decreased the level of transforming growth factor B1 (TGF-B1) and insulin like growth factor and results in the defected skull bone [23].

Dietary Fat and Bone

Several studies have been conducted to check the effect of high fat diet on bone. Most of the studies conducted on the animal showed that consumption of high fat diet induces obesity which is negatively related to the strength of bone but some contradictory studies are also available which showed that the strength of bone is determined by the fatty acid profile of fats. High fat diet induced obesity in mice decreased trabecular density which was negatively correlated with the serum leptin level. It also increased the number of adipocytes and trabecular deterioration. Neither total cholesterol nor adiponectin was correlated to bone mass. This showed that serum leptin might be thought as useful indicator for osteoporosis risk with obesity induced from diets [24]. High fat diet consumption decreases the bone formation [25]. In another study, a diet induced obesity in mice results in higher serum tartrate resistant phosphate (TRAP) and lower concentration of osteocalin. Mice fed on a higher fat diet contain less femoral bone volume connectivity density, trabecular number as compared to mice that were fed on a control diet [26]. Similarly obesity induced by short term high fat and extended high fat diets increased the cross linked telopeptides of type I collagen (CTX), insulin and leptic level which are negatively correlated with the volume and density of bone which are caused by resorption changes of trabecular architecture [27]. Similarly, another study by Genesh et al. showed a similar result that is, a decrease in bone mineral density and an increase in bone marrow adiposity, cathepsin K and cytokinesis in splenocytes and bone marrow [28]. In the same way, a study by Chen et al. showed that the consumption of high fat diets in mice increased serum non-esterified fatty acids and leptin and increased the bone resorption as compared to bone formation. It also increased bone marrow adiposity and adipogenic genes that include PPAR γ and AP_2 and decreased the osteocalcin and RunX2 which are osteoblastogenic markers [29]. Different studies related to the effect of dietary fats are summarized in Table 1.

In mice obesity induced from diets resulted in lower content of calcium and phosphorus in bone and also less weight of bone, but when these mice were fed with a diet having high fats but it contains a high amount of vitamin D and calcium (10,000 IU and 1.2% respectively), the calcium and phosphorus content of their bone was increased and also their bone weight. Consumption of a diet high in vitamin D and calcium increased the concentration of 1,25 $(OH)_2$ in blood while on the other side it decreased the osteocalcin and parathyroid hormone [19]. Consumption of a high fat diet (45%) in rat increased the concentration of serum leptin and differentiation of osteoclast resulting in reduction in the volume of trabecular bone, the number of trabecular and connectivity density. N acetylcysteine which is a precursor of glutathione, increases the concentration of glutathione resulting in less differentiation of osteoclast even though the animals are fed on a high fat diet [18]. Consumption of a fat that is either it contains saturated fatty acids, n-3 polyunsaturated fatty acids, n-6 polyunsaturated fatty acids did not affect bone mineral density of femur in rats but it affected the strength of femur bone as indicated by peak load, this is due to the fatty acids profile of femur which is determined by the fatty acid profile of the diet [30].

Table 1. Effect of dietary fat on metabolism of bone shown by different animal studies

Serial No.	Diet	Study subjects	Observed effect	Reference
1	High fat diet (60 kcal% fat)	Mice (3 week old) and Mice (15 week old) C57BL/6 male	Decrease in strength, stiffness and toughness of femoral bone in mice of both aged groups. Lowered IGF-I level in young mice only	[31]
2	High fat diet (Animal lard 18%)	Feeding to female mice C57BL/6. At the age of 10th week mating was done and feed this high fat diet was fed throughout pregnancy and lactation. Offspring fed on the same diet and sampling was done at 30th week.	High fat-fed mice offspring resulted in increased adiposity of femur, while female offspring also showed changed trabecular structure that indicates in utero programming	[32]
3	High fat diet (10% corn oil)	Fed to 12 month old female mice C57BL/6 for 6 months	Showed increased total fat mass in the body, body weight and fat mass in the abdomen while it showed decreased BMD along with increased adiposity of bone marrow and up regulation of cathepsin k, peroxisome proliferator-activated receptor γ, and increased IL-6 and tumor necrosis factor alpha in the splenocytes and bone marrow	[33]
4	Westernized diet which contains lipid 154g/kg having greater concentration of (C16:0, C18:0). Protein content of westernized diet was also less 14.3% as compared to standard which contains protein 21.4%.	Wild type OF1 female mice were fed with westernized diet just before mating and this diet was supplied during pregnancy till weaning. Offspring was fed with the same diet for 30 weeks and then sacrificed for sampling.	Showed reduced bone density and bone mineral content in the vertebral and femoral bone and in the whole body while on the other hand it showed increased adiposity and hyperinsulinemia and hypercholesterolemia.	[34]
5	Extended high fat diet (50% lipid) for 24 weeks and short term high fat i.e., for 21 week low fat (10% calories from lipid) and for 3 weeks high fat diet while the low fat diet group consumed this diet for 24 week	Seven week old C57BL/6J male mice	Obesity induced by short term high fat and extended high fat diet increased the cross linked telopeptides of type I collagen (CTX), insulin and leptic level which are negatively correlated with the volume and density of bone which are caused by resorption changes of trabecular architecture	[27]
6	Diet that is composed of laboratory chow (75%) enriched with commercial vegetable oil (15%) and skimmed milk (10%) i.e., 38.5% of diet energy is from fat source	Male Wistar rats having weight of 80 ± 6 g of 35 days old were fed with this diet "ad-libitum" for 10 weeks	Consumption of high fat showed a decrease in lean body mass and lower body mass but there was no difference in the fat mass of both lipid enriched and standard diet. BMD, skeleton area and bone mineral content was significant lower in the rats consuming lipid enriched diet.	[35]

Table 1. (Continued)

Serial No.	Diet	Study subjects	Observed effect	Reference
7	In comparison to control group diet which has 2% (w/w) lard in the high fat group diet has 19.5% (w/w) lard while another group consumed diet having high fat but it also contains 0.1% lipoic acid	C57BL/6 male mice having age of 4 week were fed with the diets for 13 week.	Bone formation was inhibited while bone resorption was increased in the high fat consuming group. IGF-I was lowered in plasma while tumor necrosis factor alpha was increased but these changes were prevented partially or completely in the group consuming diet supplemented with lipoic acid which showed that oxidation might be the mediator of bone loss through hyperlipidemia.	[36]
8	n-3 fatty acid deficient milk in which 1% fatty acid comprised of DPAn-6 or DHA%, or DHA:DPAn-6 (2:1) 1%. After 21 postnatal days the pups were fed on a diet having similar composition	Long Evans rats	The femur and tibia bone of rats consuming the DPAn-6 enriched diet have lowest BMD and BMC, while the maximum BMD and BMC were observed in DHA consuming rats which showed that DHA is an important constituent required for the development of strong bone.	[37]
9	High fat western style diet (HFWD) 20% fat from corn oil and 37.5% of total calories from fat, HFWD with mineral supplemented with the extract of *Lithothamnion calcareum* which is a rich in minerals, and low fat rodent chew diet	C57BL6/6 mice were fed with these types of diets for 15 months	Female mice consuming HFWD had less bone strength and bone mineral content as compared to low fat group and these defects were recovered in the group consuming HFWD supplemented with mineral extract. Tartrate resistant acid phosphatase (TRAP) level of serum was also higher in the group consuming a mineral supplemented diet but there was no significance difference in the markers i.e., N-terminal peptide of type I procollagen (PINP) and osteocalcin. No specific diet related effects were observed in male mice.	[38]
	Standard diet enriched with soybean oil (15%) and the other group consuming diet supplemented with sesame oil (10%)	Ovariectomized Female virgin wistar rats	Ovariectomy leads to estrogen deficiency that causes an increase in triglycerides, low density lipoprotein and total lipids in the serum along with an increase in acid phosphatase and alkaline phosphatase in urine, bone and plasma. These all parameters were improved in rats when they were fed on a diet enriched in soybean oil or sesame oil.	[39]

Dietary Protein and Bone Health

One of the important components of bone organic matrix is protein and it is required for the production of growth factor and hormones that control the synthesis of bone. Traditionally it is thought that a high intake of protein is a risk for the maintenance of bone because the consumption of protein has been shown to increase the calcium excretion through the urine [40] but some more controlled studies have shown that the consumption of low and high meat diets in post-menopausal women for a period of 8 weeks did not affect the retention of calcium or metabolism biomarkers of bone [41].

Osteoporosis caused by estrogen deficiency and the less intake of protein resulted in decreases in bone mineral density (BMD) and decreases in the strength of femur, vertebrae and tibia bone. The administration of a diet which is rich in essential amino acids increased the strength of femur, vertebrae and tibia bone and prevented further decreases in BMD. An essential amino acids supplemented diet also results in increased bone formation and a decrease in bone absorption [42]. Similarly another study showed that restricted protein supply during late pregnancy and early days of postnatal life adversely affects the growth of skeleton and metabolism of bone [43]. Another study showed that during the pregnancy maternal fat, milk and magnesium intake during the third trimester was predictive of bone mineral density of child at the age of 16 years [44].

Chronic disease of kidney results in an increase in the level of parathyroid hormone in plasma and this elevated level of parathyroid hormone is related to increased calcium resorption from bone resulting in low density as well as strength of bone [45]. Similarly chronic kidney diseases also increase the risk of osteoporosis [46]. In a mice model study uremia was caused by surgical procedure and then the mice were fed with a high soy protein diet with or without exercise and the other two groups consumed a control diet with or without exercise. At the end of study it was concluded that the consumption of the diet rich in soy protein diet along with exercise improved the relative volume of bone, number of trabecular, separation of trabecular and density of trabecular connectivity in the proximal femur [47].

A protein-rich and potential renal acid load diet increased calcium absorption from diet in postmenopausal women. The high protein and potential renal acid load diet also increased IGF-I level in serum and decreased PTH concentration in serum and did not affect bone formation and resorption biomarkers, which showed that the high protein diet not effect bone health adversely in women [48]. In contrast to this supplementation of essential amino acids in the low protein diet improved the strength of femur, vertebrae and tibia bone [42].

Dietary Vitamin D and Bone

The physiological and mechanistic perspective importance of calcium and vitamin D is well established for bone health [49, 50]. Mostly low vitamin D or calcium intake is related to higher incidence of osteopenia, hyperparathoidism and fracture of bone while higher intake of vitamin D and calcium is generally thought to be protective agents against bone diseases like osteoporosis and osteomalacia [19].

Sunlight exposure is the major source that trigger the production of Vitamin D. Change in the lifestyle and moderation have decreased the human sunshine exposure so it is need of the time to consume diets which are rich in vitamin D or fortified with vitamin D to overcome the problems of bone [51]. The dietary habits like drinking alcohol, green tea have higher bone density as compared to those having habits of cheese consumption and smoking. Since, vitamin D is a fat soluble vitamin and is readily absorbed by the fat cells so there is a correlation between obesity and vitamin D deficiency. In children the deficiency of vitamin D causes growth retardation and signs of rickets [52]. Vitamin D intoxication does not occur at concentration of 25(OH)D greater than 375 mol/L or 150 ng/L [53]. Osteoporosis and related complications prevention is an important socioeconomic priority, which necessitates the development of new nutritional approaches for osteoporosis prevention and treatment.

Vitamin D exists in two forms vitamin D_2 (ergocalciferol) and vitamin D_3 (cholcalciferol). UV radiation of sun light having wavelength of 290-315 nm converts 7 dehydrocholesterol to cholcalciferol (Vitamin D_3). In the liver 25-hydroxylase converts dietary vitamin D_3 and endogenously formed vitamin D_3 to 25 hydroxy vitamin D 25(OH)D. This 25-hydroxy vitamin is the indicator of vitamin D status. 1,25 dihydroxyvitamin D_3 is formed from 25(OH)D in the kidney and this is the active hormonal form that acts along with calcitonin and parathyroid hormone to maintain the concentration of calcium in the plasma [54]. Vitamin D is found in limited natural foods. Good sources of dietary vitamin D are oil rich fish, eggs and products that are fortified like margarine, breakfast cereals and reduced fat spreads [55].

As described earlier the deficiency of vitamin D leads to osteomalacia, a defect in bone mineralization and also leads to hypophosphatemia, hypocalcemia and hyperthyroidism [56]. Similarly a study was conducted to investigate the relationship of vitamin D and calcium deficiency on osteoporosis, varied concentration of vitamin D and calcium were fed to adult female rats. Rats were divided into two groups i.e., a diet deficient in vitamin D and a replete diet and then further provided either 0.1% or 1% calcium in the diet for 3 months. 25-hydroxyvitamin D (25D) level was found to be 14 nmol/L in the vitamin D deplete group while those fed with replete vitamin D was found to have 97-135 nmol/L (25 D) concentration. Osteoid maturation time (OMT) was found to be 6 days in vitamin D replete diet as compared to vitamin D deplete 0.1% calcium diet having OMT of 12.6 days. This results in diagnostic for osteomalacia. Cortical width and metaphyseal trabecular bone volume were found to be less in vitamin D replete and 0.1% calcium, and vitamin D deficient and 1% calcium as compared to vitamin D replete having 1% calcium. So osteomalacia is caused when both vitamin D and calcium are deficient while deficiency of calcium alone or low vitamin D status in osteoporosis when adequate dietary calcium is taken results [57].

Low concentration of 25-hydroxyvitamin D in pregnant women was not associated with the length of fetal femur but it was correlated with metaphyseal area of femur and greater femoral splayine index that is a ratio of metaphyseal cross sectional area of femur to length of femur in gestation 19th week. This shows that vitamin D status during early pregnancy should be instituted to better development of femur [58].

HORMONE

Mineral metabolism in man is controlled by five important hormones which include parathyroid hormone, vitamin D and corresponding molecules, fibroblast growth factor 23, peptides related to parathyroid hormone and calcitonin. Some other hormones like androgen, estrogen, growth hormone and cortisol modify the effect of above major hormones [59].

Parathyroid hormone affects bone by two ways i.e., under normal condition bone formation is promoted through a receptor which is present in osteoblast, while under hypocalcemia condition bone resorption is stimulated by PTH from the bone which is larger reservoir of calcium so that normal calcaemia condition might be restored. Osteoclasts have very limited receptors for PTH and resorption of bone is due to changes in osteoclast and osteoblast relationship. Osteoblast produces receptor activator of nuclear factor kappa-B ligand (RANKL) and osteoprotegrin. Differentiation of osteoclast is stimulated by RANKL, while osteoprotegrin controls the action of RNKL by inhibiting its activity. Parathyroid like peptides or substances have same biological activity but their immunological effects are different. C cells of thyroid gland produce calcitonin. In contrast to PTH calcitonin is secreted due to high level of calcium in plasma (hypercalcemia) [60]. Function of calcitonin is to reduce the level of calcium in the plasma [61].

CALCIUM INTAKE AND BONE HEALTH

About 1200 g of calcium is present in an adult of which 99% calcium is found in the bone while the remaining part of calcium is found in circulating plasma or intracellular cationic form [61]. Calcium is an important mineral which is required for the normal development of bone and skeleton [62]. So sufficient intake of calcium is required for acquiring optimum peak bone mass and it also affects subsequent bone loss due to aging. Less intake of calcium leads to hyperthyroidism and consequently leads to resorption of bone. Beside from sufficient intake of calcium, the absorption of calcium from diets is an important factor which determines the availability of calcium for the maintenance and development of skeleton. Therefore it is required that other food components are to be identified which positively or negatively affect the absorption of calcium [63]. In food calcium is found as salts or calcium ions complexes with other dietary components. Thus calcium must be released from these complexes and made it into soluble form i.e., ionized form so that it can be absorbed. In soluble form calcium is absorbed by paracellular and transcellular pathways [64]. Calbinidin (D9k) is a crystalline protein that binds to calcium and helps in intracellular diffusion of calcium ions, while biosynthesis of calbinidin is dependent upon the availability of vitamin D. So people who are deficient in vitamin D may suffer from calcium deficiency even though their intake of calcium is high. Among other food components that promote the absorption of calcium are components of milk like casein phosphopeptides, lactulose and lactose. Similarly oligosaccharides that are not digestible also increase calcium absorption [65]. But in contrast to calcium less intake of sodium 2g/day in postmenopausal women for 6 months resulted in significant decreases in the excretion of calcium and sodium and bone turnover markers, but it did not affect parathyroid hormone or 1,25 dihydroxyvitamin [66].

MAGNESIUM

Low concentration of magnesium in the plasma leads to hypocalcemia which in turn stimulates the release of calcium from bone. Hypocalcemia is low concentration of magnesium because magnesium is required for the secretion of parathyroid hormone and PTH receptor activation by ligand. Low concentration of magnesium in plasma might be due to low dietary intake of magnesium, less absorption of magnesium from intensity and other factors that result in excessive magnesium leakage from renal tubule [67].

PHOSPHORUS AND BONE

Phosphorus is an important component of bone minerals. Deficiency of phosphorus results in impaired bone mineralization. However there is little evidence which showed the phosphorus related osteoporosis incidence but on the other hand if a diet is rich in phosphorus and deficient in calcium it increases the level of parathyroid hormone after four weeks in young adults. Consumption of carbonated beverages which are rich in phosphorus has resulted in more fractures and less bone mass in adults. Nutritional recommendation of phosphorus varies for different age groups, i.e., for adolescence 1250 mg/d, for adults 700 mg/d and for people over the age of 50 years 580 mg/d, and the phosphate level of serum is directly influenced by dietary phosphorus intake [68].

DIETARY ZINC AND BONE

Zinc is an important mineral for the development of healthy bone. Zinc deficiency is associated with retarded bone growth [69]. A large proportion of body zinc is found in bone and it has been shown that it concentrates in the osteoid layer before calcification. Since bone is a sink of zinc so breakdown of skeleton results in a release of zinc and it is mostly reabsorbed for skeleton development [69].

Zinc affects skeleton by two ways, i.e., an increase in bone formation by stimulation of osteoblast and a decrease in bone resorption by inhibiting osteoclasts. Calvaria cultured on Dulbecco's modified eagle medium showed greater uptake of zinc by increasing the concentration of zinc in the medium. In bone tissue the activity of ATPase was increased by zinc but it did not affect the pyrophosphatase and B-N-acetylglucosaminidase activity [70]. Similarly culturing in zinc medium also increased collagen content. Proliferation and differentiation of osteoblast are stimulated by zinc containing medium. When osteoblastic MC3T3-E1 cells were grown in zinc containing medium DNA, cell proliferation was activated, protein synthesis was inhibited and stimulation of osteoblast was blocked, which suggest that zinc stimulation activity might be dependent on synthesis of protein.

Patients having osteoporosis have low zinc level in the skeleton as compared to control, and in postmenopausal women zinc concentration in the urine is an indicator of resorption of bone and women having osteoporosis excrete more than 800 μg/g creatinine in urine. Supplementation of trace minerals have been shown to increase the bone mineral density [71]. In Vitro it has been shown that resorption of bone by osteoclast is inhibited by zinc. When calaria cells of rats were grown in medium containing PTH, interleukin-Ia prostaglandian E2 and lipopolysaccharides, they decreased the bone calcium content, but this decrease in bone calcium content was completely inhibited when zinc was added to the medium [72].

POSTMENOPAUSAL OSTEOPOROSIS PREVENTION BY PHYTOESTROGENS

Estrogen plays an important role in the maintenance of bone health by increasing the apoptosis of osteoclast and decreasing cytokines that promote the activity of osteoclast. So the deficiency of estrogen increases the loss of bone at every stage of life. Similarly the deficiency of estrogen decreases the osteoblast life spam of osteoclast so resulting in the loss of bone [73]. Phytoestrogen can be defined as compounds derived from plant and that are able to generate estrogenic response in the body [74]. A large number of phytoestrogen are found in the plant and can be divided into many classes, but the important ones that are useful for men are isoflavones and lignans [75].

The deficiency of estrogen is a major factor contributing to the incidence of osteoporosis in women. Hormone replacement therapy (HRT) is used to minimize bone loss in postmenopausal women. But due to less uptake and side effects of HRT that it could cause malignancy, researches have been focused towards the dietary phytoestrogens that are naturally found in the plant and are non-steroidal, which resemble the natural estrogen in structure and can bind with estrogen receptors [76]. Mechanism of action of phytoestrogen on bone health has been elucidated in Figure 1.

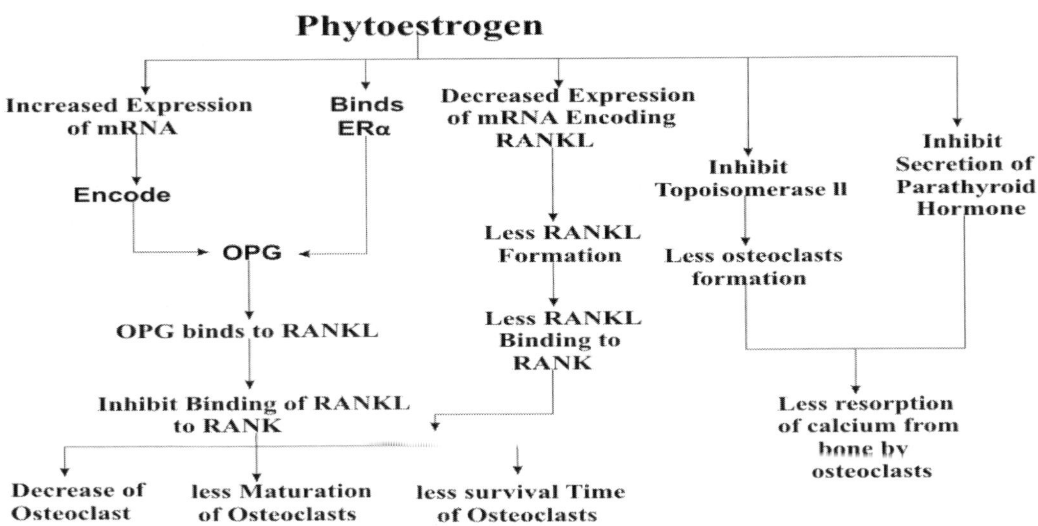

Figure 1. Mechanism of action of Phytoestrogen on turnover.

Morabito showed that genistein which is an isoflavone found in soy, consumption of 56 mg/d and hormonal replacement therapy for 12 months increased BMD significantly in the lumber spine and femur. Similar results were observed for both hormonal therapy and genistein so osteoporosis caused by estrogen deficiency can be recovered by consuming phytoestrogen [77]. But genistein concentration found in the natural food is much low and this level of genistein can be achieved by supplementation or functional food development.

Consumption of fructooligosaccharides enhanced isoflavones protective effects on the skeleton. Increasing consumption of isoflavones 10, 20, 40, 80 μg/g body weight enhanced significantly bone mineral density as well as bone strength. When these rats were fed with fructooligosaccharides the protective effect of isoflavones 10 μg/g was maximized to the extent similar to 80 μg/g. So fructooligosacharides enhance the effect of isoflavones by acting as prebiotic [78].

Isoflavones are mostly found in the family fabaceae that include peanut, soy and clover. Family euphorniaceae and iridiaceae are also good source of isoflavones. A soy based diet either it is fermented or non-fermented is the major source of isoflavones [79, 80]. Good sources of lignans are whole grain, flaxseed, tea, vegetables and berries. Among these sources flaxseed is the richest source of lignin having 0.96-3.15 μmol lignin/g [81].

Prevention of Bone Diseases

An addition of phytase in diets results in an increase in body weight and bone mineral content. This is done to improve the Zn status because phytic acid binds with nutritionally important minerals like Zn. So the addition of phytase removes these minerals from phytic acid thus making them bioavailable. The addition of phytase in diets results in an increase in the mass of tibia and femur and makes them stronger [82]. Drinking of deep sea water along with exercise prevents osteoporosis and increases peak bone mass in rats. This is due to the fact that deep sea water is rich in Mg^{+2}, Ca^{+2}, and K^{+} [83]. The addition of selenium or selenium plus iodine in the diet of rats results in chrondrocytes diminished necrosis and volume of bone in comparison to volume and tissue, thickness of trabecular and trabecular number increased, while decreases in trabecular separation. So a Kashin-Beck diseases (KBD) endemic area diet feeding to rats results in necrosis of chondrocytes and impairments in bone development [84].

Among popular beverages, green tea is one of them. Several studies had shown that green tea consumption helps in the loss of body weight [85, 86]. These anti-obestic effects of green tea are due to higher fat oxidation and thermogenesis and decreased peroxidation of lipids [87]. The extract of green tea which is rich in poly phenolic had been found to be osteoprotective [88]. The consumption of green tea polyphenols (0.5) in drinking water of mice increased the fat free mass and strength of bone while on the other hand it also decreased the markers of bone turn over which include leptin, serum insulin like growth factor I, proinflamatory cytokines and adiponectin [89].

Conclusion

Due to less effectiveness of treatment for degenerative diseases and side effects of drugs like hormone replacement therapy for bone diseases of postmenopausal women it is better to consider preventive approach for these diseases. In the prevention of these diseases a diet plays an important role because certain dietary habits like vegetarian diet and Westernized diet i.e., more intake of fat especially vegetable fat makes the people at more risks for bone diseases. So a healthy diet which includes consumption of fruits, vegetables, proteins and fat from different sources helps in the prevention of bone diseases. Another important factor is that the maternal dietary habits that affect the skeleton of offspring, so pregnant women should consume a diet which is rich in minerals and healthy fat and protein that are rich in essential amino acids. Another important aspect of diets for bone diseases is the development of functional food which is rich in isoflavones can be an effective alternative for hormone replacement therapy of osteoporotic women.

REFERENCES

[1] Morris HA, O'Loughlin PD, Anderson PH. Experimental evidence for the effects of calcium and vitamin D on bone: a review. *Nutrients* 2010; 2(9):1026-1035.

[2] Weaver CM. The growing years and prevention of osteoporosis in later life. *Proc. Nutr. Soc.* 2000; 59(02):303-306.

[3] Rowling MJ, Gliniak C, Welsh J, Fleet JC. High dietary vitamin D prevents hypocalcemia and osteomalacia in CYP27B1 knockout mice. *J. Nutr.* 2007; 137(12):2608-2615.

[4] Cooper C, Melton LJ. Epidemiology of osteoporosis. *Trends Endocrinol. Metab.* 1992;3(6):224-229.

[5] Bonjour JP, Schurch MA, Rizzoli R. Nutritional aspects of hip fractures. *Bone.* 1996;18(3):139-144.

[6] Yamaguchi M. Regulatory mechanism of food factors in bone metabolism and prevention of osteoporosis. *Yakugaku Zasshi.* 2006;126(11):1117-1137.

[7] Hoppe C, Mølgaard C, Michaelsen KF. Bone size and bone mass in 10-year-old Danish children: effect of current diet. *Osteoporos Int.* 2000;11(12):1024-1030.

[8] Bass EF, Baile CA, Lewis RD, Giraudo SQ. Bone quality and strength are greater in growing male rats fed fructose compared with glucose. *Nutr. Res.* 2013;33(12):1063-1071.

[9] Smith AM. Veganism and osteoporosis: a review of the current literature. *Int. J. Nurs. Pract.* 2006;12(5):302-306.

[10] Heaney R, Abrams S, Dawson-Hughes B, Looker A, Marcus R, Matkovic V, et al. Peak bone mass. *Osteoporos Int.* 2000;11(12):985-1009.

[11] Turner-McGrievy GM, Barnard ND, Scialli AR, Lanou AJ. Effects of a low-fat vegan diet and a Step II diet on macro-and micronutrient intakes in overweight postmenopausal women. *Nutr.* 2004;20(9):738 746.

[12] Gjesdal CG, Vollset SE, Ueland PM, Refsum H, Meyer HE, Tell GS. Plasma homocysteine, folate, and vitamin B12 and the risk of hip fracture: the Hordaland Homocysteine Study. *J. Bone Miner Res.* 2007;22(5):747-756.

[13] Krivosikova Z, Krajcovicova-Kudlackova M, Spustova V, Stefikova K, Valachovicova M, Blazicek P, et al. The association between high plasma homocysteine levels and lower bone mineral density in Slovak women: the impact of vegetarian diet. *Eur J. Nutr.* 2010;49(3):147-153.

[14] Shoelson SE, Herrero L, Naaz A. Obesity, inflammation, and insulin resistance. *Gastroenterol.* 2007; 132(6):2169-2180.

[15] Furukawa S, Fujita T, Shimabukuro M, Iwaki M, Yamada Y, Nakajima Y, et al. Increased oxidative stress in obesity and its impact on metabolic syndrome. *J. Clin. Invest.* 2004;114(12):1752.

[16] Rosen CJ, Bouxsein ML. Mechanisms of disease: is osteoporosis the obesity of bone? *Nat. Clin. Pract. Rheumatol.* 2006;2(1):35-43.

[17] Zhao LJ, Liu YJ, Liu PY, Hamilton J, Recker RR, Deng H-W. Relationship of obesity with osteoporosis. *J. Clin. Endocrinol. Metab.* 2007;92(5):1640-1646.

[18] Cao JJ, Picklo MJ. N-acetylcysteine supplementation decreases osteoclast differentiation and increases bone mass in mice fed a high-fat diet. *J. Nutr.* 2014;144(3):289-296.

[19] Song Q, Sergeev IN. High vitamin D and calcium intakes increase bone mineral (Ca and P) content in high-fat diet-induced obese mice. *Nutr. Res.* 2015;35(2):146-154 doi: 10.1016/j.nutres.2014.11.003.

[20] Boeing H, Bechthold A, Bub A, Ellinger S, Haller D, Kroke A, et al. Critical review: vegetables and fruit in the prevention of chronic diseases. *Eur. J. Nutr.* 2012;51(6):637-663.

[21] Weinstein RS. Glucocorticoid-induced bone disease. *N. Engl. J. Med.* 2011;365(1):62-70.

[22] Livingstone DEW, Jones GC, Smith K, Jamieson PM, Andrew R, Kenyon CJ, et al. Understanding the Role of Glucocorticoids in Obesity: Tissue-Specific Alterations of Corticosterone Metabolism in Obese Zucker Rats. *Endocrinol.* 2000;141(2):560-563.

[23] Santoso MI, Rohman MS. Decreased TGF-beta1 and IGF-1 protein expression in rat embryo skull bone in folic acid-restricted diet. *J Nutr. Biochem.* 2006;17(1):51-56.

[24] Fujita Y, Watanabe K, Maki K. Serum leptin levels negatively correlate with trabecular bone mineral density in high-fat diet-induced obesity mice. *J. Musculoskelet Neuronal Interact.* 2012; 12(2):84-94.

[25] Tagliaferri C, Salles J, Landrier JF, Giraudet C, Patrac V, Lebecque P, et al. Increased body fat mass and tissue lipotoxicity associated with ovariectomy or high-fat diet differentially affects bone and skeletal muscle metabolism in rats. *Eur. J. Nutr.* 2014.

[26] Cao JJ, Sun L, Gao H. Diet-induced obesity alters bone remodeling leading to decreased femoral trabecular bone mass in mice. *Ann. NY Acad. Sci.* 2010;1192(1):292-297.

[27] Patsch JM, Kiefer FW, Varga P, Pail P, Rauner M, Stupphann D, et al. Increased bone resorption and impaired bone microarchitecture in short-term and extended high-fat diet–induced obesity. *Metab.* 2011;60(2):243-249.

[28] Halade GV, Rahman MM, Williams PJ, Fernandes G. High fat diet-induced animal model of age-associated obesity and osteoporosis. *J. Nutr. Biochem.* 2010;21(12):1162-1169.

[29] Chen JR, Lazarenko OP, Wu X, Tong Y, Blackburn ML, Shankar K, et al. Obesity reduces bone density associated with activation of PPARgamma and suppression of Wnt/beta-catenin in rapidly growing male rats. *PLoS One.* 2010;5(10):0013704.

[30] Lau BY, Fajardo VA, McMeekin L, Sacco SM, Ward WE, Roy BD, et al. Influence of high-fat diet from differential dietary sources on bone mineral density, bone strength,

and bone fatty acid composition in rats. *Appl. Physiol. Nutr. Metab.* 2010;35(5):598-606.
[31] Ionova-Martin SS, Wade JM, Tang S, Shahnazari M, Ager JW, 3rd, Lane NE, et al. Changes in cortical bone response to high-fat diet from adolescence to adulthood in mice. *Osteoporos Int.* 2011;22(8):2283-2293.
[32] Lanham SA, Roberts C, Hollingworth T, Sreekumar R, Elahi MM, Cagampang FR, et al. Maternal high-fat diet: effects on offspring bone structure. *Osteoporos Int.* 2010;21(10):1703-1714.
[33] Halade GV, Rahman MM, Williams PJ, Fernandes G. High fat diet-induced animal model of age-associated obesity and osteoporosis. *J. Nutr. Biochem.* 2010;21(12):1162-1169.
[34] Demigne C, Bloch-Faure M, Picard N, Sabboh H, Besson C, Remesy C, et al. Mice chronically fed a westernized experimental diet as a model of obesity, metabolic syndrome and osteoporosis. *Eur. J. Nutr.* 2006;45(5):298-306.
[35] Lac G, Cavalie H, Ebal E, Michaux O. Effects of a high fat diet on bone of growing rats. Correlations between visceral fat, adiponectin and bone mass density. *Lipids Health Dis.* 2008;7(1):16.
[36] Xiao Y, Cui J, Li YX, Shi YH, Wang B, Le GW, et al. Dyslipidemic high-fat diet affects adversely bone metabolism in mice associated with impaired antioxidant capacity. *Nutr.* 2011;27(2):214-220.
[37] Li Y, Seifert MF, Lim SY, Salem N, Watkins BA. Bone mineral content is positively correlated to n-3 fatty acids in the femur of growing rats. *Br. J. Nutr.* 2010;104(05):674-685.
[38] Aslam MN, Kreider JM, Paruchuri T, Bhagavathula N, DaSilva M, Zernicke RF, et al. A mineral-rich extract from the red marine algae Lithothamnion calcareum preserves bone structure and function in female mice on a Western-style diet. *Calcif Tissue Int.* 2010;86(4):313-324.
[39] Hassan HA, Wakf AME, Gharib NEE. Role of phytoestrogenic oils in alleviating osteoporosis associated with ovariectomy in rats. *Cytotechnol.* 2013;65(4):609-619.
[40] Feskanich D, Willett WC, Stampfer MJ, Colditz GA. Protein consumption and bone fractures in women. *Am J Epidemiol.* 1996; 143(5):472-479.
[41] Roughead ZKF, Johnson LK, Lykken GI, Hunt JR. Controlled high meat diets do not affect calcium retention or indices of bone status in healthy postmenopausal women. *J. Nutr.* 2003;133 (4):1020-1026.
[42] Ammann P, Laib A, Bonjour JP, Meyer J, Rüegsegger P, Rizzoli R. Dietary Essential Amino Acid Supplements Increase Bone Strength by Influencing Bone Mass and Bone Microarchitecture in Ovariectomized Adult Rats Fed an Isocaloric Low-Protein Diet. *J. Bone Miner Res.* 2002;17(7):1264-1272.
[43] Fetoui H, Mahjoubi-Samet A, Guermazi F, Zeghal N. Maternal low-protein diet affects bone mass and mineral metabolism in suckling rats. *J Anim. Physiol. Anim. Nutr. (Berl).* 2008;92(4):448-455.
[44] Yin J, Dwyer T, Riley M, Cochrane J, Jones G. The association between maternal diet during pregnancy and bone mass of the children at age 16. *Eur. J. Clin. Nutr.* 2010;64(2):131-137.
[45] Moe SM, Drüeke T. Improving global outcomes in mineral and bone disorders. *Clinical Journal of the American Society of Nephrology.* 2008; 3 (Supplement 3):S127-S130.

[46] Doherty TM, Fitzpatrick LA, Inoue D, Qiao JH, Fishbein MC, Detrano RC, et al. Molecular, endocrine, and genetic mechanisms of arterial calcification. *Endocr. Rev.* 2004;25(4):629-672.

[47] Tomayko EJ, Chung HR, Wilund KR. Soy protein diet and exercise training increase relative bone volume and enhance bone microarchitecture in a mouse model of uremia. *J. Bone Miner Metab.* 2011;29(6):682-690.

[48] Cao JJ, Johnson LK, Hunt JR. A diet high in meat protein and potential renal acid load increases fractional calcium absorption and urinary calcium excretion without affecting markers of bone resorption or formation in postmenopausal women. *J. Nutr.* 2011;141(3):391-397.

[49] Christakos S, Hewison M, Gardner DG, Wagner CL, Sergeev IN, Rutten E, et al. Vitamin D: beyond bone. *Ann. N Y Acad. Sci.* 2013;1287(1):45-58.

[50] Sergeev IN. Vitamin D and cellular Ca^{2+} signaling in breast cancer. *Anticancer Res.* 2012;32(1):299-302.

[51] Holick MF, Chen TC. Vitamin D deficiency: a worldwide problem with health consequences. *Am. J. Clin. Nutr.* 2008;87(4):1080S-1086S.

[52] Dawson-Hughes B, Heaney RP, Holick MF, Lips P, Meunier PJ, Vieth R. Estimates of optimal vitamin D status. *Osteoporosis Int.* 2005;16(7):713-716.

[53] Holick MF. Vitamin D deficiency. *N. Engl. J. Med.* 2007;357(3):266-281.

[54] O'Connor A, Benelam B. An update on UK Vitamin D intakes and status, and issues for food fortification and supplementation. *Nutr. Bull.* 2011;36(3):390-396.

[55] Vieth R. Vitamin D supplementation, 25-hydroxyvitamin D concentrations, and safety. *Am. J. Clin. Nutr.* 1999;69(5):842-856.

[56] Underwood JL, DeLuca HF. Vitamin D is not directly necessary for bone growth and mineralization. *Am. J. Physiol-Endocrinol Met.* 1984;246(6):E493-E498.

[57] Morris HA, O'loughlin PD, Anderson PH. Experimental evidence for the effects of calcium and vitamin D on bone: a review. *Nutrients.* 2010;2(9):1026-1035.

[58] Mahon P, Harvey N, Crozier S, Inskip H, Robinson S, Arden N, et al. Low maternal vitamin D status and fetal bone development: cohort study. *J. Bone Miner Res.* 2010;25(1):14-19.

[59] Allgrove J. Voyages of Discovery. *Endocr. Dev.* 2009;16:1-7.

[60] Allgrove J, Adami S, Manning R, O'Riordan J. Cytochemical bioassay of parathyroid hormone in maternal and cord blood. *Arch. Dis. Child.* 1985;60(2):110-115.

[61] Allgrove J. Physiology of calcium, phosphate and magnesium. *Endocr. Dev.* 2009:8-31.

[62] Medicine IO. Dietary Reference Intakes for Calcium, Phosphorus, Magnesium, Vitamin D, and Fluoride. Washington, DC: The National Academies Press; 1997. 448 p.

[63] Cashman K. Calcium intake, calcium bioavailability and bone health. *Br. J. Nutr.* 2002; 87(2):169-178.

[64] Cashman K. Prebiotics and calcium bioavailability. *Curr. Issues Intestinal Microbiol.* 2003; 4(1):21-32.

[65] Cashman KD. A prebiotic substance persistently enhances intestinal calcium absorption and increases bone mineralization in young adolescents. *Nutr. Rev.* 2006;64(4):189-196.

[66] Carbone LD, Barrow KD, Bush AJ, Boatright MD, Michelson JA, Pitts KA, et al. Effects of a low sodium diet on bone metabolism. *J. Bone Miner Metab.* 2005;23(6):506-513.

[67] Shaw N. A practical approach to hypocalcaemia in children. *Endocr. Dev.* 2009;16:73-92.
[68] Palacios C. The role of nutrients in bone health, from A to Z. *Crit. Rev. Food Sci. Nutr.* 2006;46(8):621-628.
[69] Yamaguchi M. Nutritional factors and bone homeostasis: synergistic effect with zinc and genistein in osteogenesis. *Mol. Cell Biochem.* 2012;366(1-2):201-221.
[70] Yamaguchi M, Oishi H, Suketa Y. Zinc stimulation of bone protein synthesis in tissue culture: activation of aminoacyl-tRNA synthetase. *Biochem. Pharmacol.* 1988;37(21):4075-4080.
[71] Reginster JY, Strause L, Saltman P, Franchimont P. Trace elements and postmenopausal osteoporosis: a preliminary report of decreased serum manganese. *Med. Sci. Res.* 1988;16:337-338.
[72] Yamaguchi M, Segawa Y, Shimokawa N, Tsuzuike N, Tagashira E. Inhibitory Effect of β-Alanyl-L-Histidinato Zinc on Bone Resorption in Tissue Culture. *Pharmacol.* 1992;45(5):292-300.
[73] Chiechi LM, Micheli L. Utility of dietary phytoestrogens in preventing postmenopausal osteoporosis. *Curr. Top Nutrceut. Res.* 2005;3(1):15-28.
[74] Adlercreutz H. Phytoestrogens. State of the art. *Environ Toxicol Pharmacol.* 1999;7(3):201-207.
[75] Adlercreutz H. Phytoestrogens and Cancer. *Lancet Oncol.* 2002;3:364-373.
[76] Cotter A, Cashman KD. Genistein appears to prevent early postmenopausal bone loss as effectively as hormone replacement therapy. *Nutr Rev.* 2003;61(10):346-351.
[77] Morabito N, Crisafulli A, Vergara C, Gaudio A, Lasco A, Frisina N, et al. Effects of Genistein and Hormone-Replacement Therapy on Bone Loss in Early Postmenopausal Women: A Randomized Double-Blind Placebo-Controlled Study. *J. Bone Miner Res.* 2002;17(10):1904-1912.
[78] Mathey J, Puel C, Kati-Coulibaly S, Bennetau–Pelissero C, Davicco M, Lebecque P, et al. Fructooligosaccharides maximize bone-sparing effects of soy isoflavone-enriched diet in the ovariectomized rat. *Calcif. Tissue Int.* 2004;75(2):169-179.
[79] Ososki AL, Kennelly EJ. Phytoestrogens: a review of the present state of research. *Phytother Res.* 2003;17(8):845-869.
[80] Ahmad A, Kaleem M, Ahmed Z, Shafiq H. Therapeutic Potential of Flavonoids and Their Mechanism of Action against Microbial and Viral Infections-A Review. *Food Res Int.* 2015.
[81] Cornwell T, Cohick W, Raskin I. Dietary phytoestrogens and health. *Phytochemistry.* 2004;65(8):995-1016.
[82] McClung JP, Stahl CH, Marchitelli LJ, Morales-Martinez N, Mackin KM, Young AJ, et al. Effects of dietary phytase on body weight gain, body composition and bone strength in growing rats fed a low-zinc diet. *J. Nutr. Biochem.* 2006;17(3):190-196.
[83] Kang J, Kwon D, Park J, Shin YO, Lee JB, Igawa S, et al. Deep-sea water supplementation and swimming exercise improves bone metabolism in growing rats fed a high-fat diet. *Food Sci. Biotechnol.* 2011;20(3):665-670.
[84] Yao Y, Pei F, Li X, Yang J, Shen B, Zhou Z, et al. Preventive effects of supplemental selenium and selenium plus iodine on bone and cartilage development in rats fed with diet from Kashin–Beck disease endemic area. *Biolog Trace Element Res.* 2012;146(2):199-206.

[85] Hsu CH, Tsai T-H, Kao YH, Hwang KC, Tseng TY, Chou P. Effect of green tea extract on obese women: a randomized, double-blind, placebo-controlled clinical trial. *Clin. Nutr.* 2008;27(3):363-370.

[86] Wang H, Wen Y, Du Y, Yan X, Guo H, Rycroft JA, et al. Effects of catechin enriched green tea on body composition. *Obesity.* 2010;18(4):773-779.

[87] Basu A, Sanchez K, Leyva MJ, Wu M, Betts NM, Aston CE, et al. Green tea supplementation affects body weight, lipids, and lipid peroxidation in obese subjects with metabolic syndrome. *J. Am. Coll. Nutr.* 2010;29(1):31-40.

[88] Shen CL, Yeh JK, Cao JJ, Chyu MC, Wang JS. Green tea and bone health: evidence from laboratory studies. *Pharmacol. Res.* 2011;64(2):155-161.

[89] Shen CL, Cao JJ, Dagda RY, Chanjaplammootil S, Lu C, Chyu MC, et al. Green tea polyphenols benefits body composition and improves bone quality in long-term high-fat diet–induced obese rats. *Nutr. Res.* 2012;32(6):448-457.

In: Diets and Diseases: Causes and Prevention
Editor: Wenbiao Wu
ISBN: 978-1-63484-580-9

Chapter 8

Diet and Arthritis: Causes, Prevention and Treatment

Oluwatoyin Bolanle Oluwole**, Adesioye Temiloluwa, Owolabi Samuel, Kosoko Babatunde and Agboola Bukola
Department of Food Technology,
Federal Institute of Industrial Research, Oshodi, Lagos, Nigeria

Abstract

A detailed review of arthritis and its various forms, causes and symptoms is reported in this chapter. Diets that trigger arthritis are discussed, and diets that could help to prevent and manage arthritis, in addition to weight loss as well as physical exercises around the joints, are proposed. Increasing daily consumption of antioxidant rich food and processed food products is suggested in preventing and managing arthritis.

Keywords: arthritis, diet, trigger, exercise, antioxidant, food

Introduction

Arthritis is the inflammation of the joints in one or more areas of the body [1]. There are several types of arthritis and they all have different symptoms, causes and treatment methods. Symptoms of arthritis may occur gradually, however, some may occur unexpectedly. Arthritis is a disease common in adults above 65 years although it could also occur in children and teens [2]. Arthritis is also more common among adults who are obese than among those who are of normal weight or underweight.

* Corresponding Author address: Department of Food Technology, Federal Institute of Industrial Research, Oshodi, Lagos, Nigeria. Email: oluwatoyinoluwole575@yahoo.com.

Osteoarthritis is one of the most common forms of arthritis caused by normal decline in the effectiveness of body function as one ages [1]. The history of developing osteoarthritis may be higher if there is an existing family history of the disease [2].

According to the Centre of Disease Control and Prevention, in overweight persons arthritis is prevalent in women than in men [3]. Arthritis can be managed by improving and consuming a healthy diet, maintaining moderate weight and carrying out physical activities regularly. In this chapter, the relationship between diet and arthritis will be further detailed.

EPIDEMIOLOGY

Generally, arthritis affects about 0.5-1% of the population all over the world. In the United Kingdom, the prevalence of rheumatoid arthritis (RA) is about 0.8% which is approximately about 400,000 people from amongst the population. The incidence rate in female is about 4 times more than that of male which indicates that women are more susceptible to RA than men although both genders could develop it [4]. However, RA has a variable estimated prevalence in developing countries. In countries like Nigeria, Indonesia and Africa generally studies have shown a lower prevalence of RA than those reported from the western countries [5].

In Canada, about 16% of people over the age of 15 years suffer from one form of arthritis or the other. Every year in Canada about 100,000 Canadians are diagnosed with arthritis, and about 1 in 1000 children are diagnosed for juvenile arthritis. In the United States about 27 million adults are affected by osteoarthritis and this is the most common cause of disability amongst them. The United States has a high prevalence rate of arthritis which could increase in 2030 to about 67 million people amongst the adult population if not properly checked [2].

TYPES OF ARTHRITIS

Arthritis occurs in different forms, it could be an inflammatory arthritis which causes pain, swelling, stiffness and fatigue. The most common cause of arthritis is osteoarthritis, this occurs from the breakage of the bone cartilage which causes pain and stiffness when they rub against each other. Osteoarthritis is common at the spine, hips, ankles and knees which are all weight bearing joints. Obesity, previous injury, traumatic situations, estrogen use, nutrition and genetic factors could cause osteoarthritis, which makes it a multifactorial disease [1].

Rheumatoid arthritis (RA) is the second most common form of arthritis which is caused by an inflammation of the joints at the synovium that occur mainly in the hands and feet. Risk factors associated with RA may include those with a family history of rheumatoid, babies born overweight who could eventually develop this defect in the future, the environment, the female gender and also those who smoke. RA occurs between the ages of 45-65 and it is most common in the female gender than in the male gender [4].

And another form of osteoarthritis is gout; it occurs when there is an accumulation of uric acid in form of crystal like deposits at the joints which causes inflammation. It occurs commonly at the wrist and knees. Other forms of arthritis include infectious arthritis which is caused by a bacterial, fungal or viral infection, this causes joint destruction and fever.

Juvenile rheumatoid arthritis is another form of arthritis that occurs in children under the age of sixteen it causes discomfort in the body through swellings in the knees, elbow and shoulders, fever and chilly feelings, pain and body rash. Psoriatic arthritis occurs at the joints of the fingers and toes causing swellings and red scaly patches around the elbows and neck. It is common in people with psoriasis.

Fibromyalgia is another form of arthritis that occurs at tender points of the body hereby causing aches, it occurs especially at shoulder, hips, arms, neck, bag and legs with symptoms such as stiffness, fatigue, headaches and muscle pain.

Systemic Lupus Erythematosus is another form of arthritis that damages healthy cells and tissues thereby causing damage to the brain, skin, joints, blood vessels, heart and lungs. It comes with symptoms such as facial rash, pain, swelling and fatigue.

Causes of Arthritis

Cartilage is a flexible connective tissue in the joint that absorbs the pressure and shock created from motion such as like during running and walking. It also cushions the joints and enables easy movement. Some forms of arthritis are caused by a reduction in the normal functioning of the cartilage tissue. However, osteoarthritis can be aggravated by an infection or injury to the joints. This occurs when the cartilage loses its cushioning ability around the bones hereby making the bones susceptible to sliding from their normal position and this causes pain and stiffness. Osteoarthritis is often referred to as the "degenerative joint disease" because of the breakdown of cartilage in the joints [6].

Rheumatoid arthritis (RA) is another form of arthritis which occurs when the body's tissues (synovium) are attacked by the immune system. The synovium, secretes a fluid that nourishes the cartilage and lubricates the joints. Therefore this may finally lead to the destruction of both the bone and cartilage inside the joint.

Pathophysiology of Arthritis

Rheumatoid arthritis is a chronic inflammatory disease that induces joint pain. It causes the weakening of bones which leads to osteoporosis which is a major cause of fracture. RA poses an increased risk of cardiovascular disease and at other times premature death as a result of the damage which occurs from its aetiology [6].

As a result of joint pains caused by inflammation the ability to engage in physical activities becomes diminished and this affects human fitness. RA is associated with other comorbid diseases such as hypertension, asthma, chronic obstructive pulmonary disease (COPD), diabetes mellitus, tuberculosis and chronic liver disease amongst other diseases [6].

Osteoarthritis is associated with soft articular cartilage which becomes inflamed thereby reducing its ability to withstand any load thus gradually the joint space becomes thinner and with time sclerosis and osteophytes occurs in the subchondral bones. Gout is another form of arthritis that occurs in the tarsometatarsal joints of the big toe and this is the major first symptom of this type of arthritis [6].

Signs of Arthritis

The most common symptoms of arthritis involve the joints. Joint pain and stiffness are typical signs along with the swelling of the joints and redness of the skin around the joint. Severe rheumatoid arthritis can cause joint deformity if left untreated. Osteoarthritis has distinct symptoms such as morning stiffness lasting for about 60 minutes, increased pain with increased weight and activity and locking of joints [2]. Gout could be acute or chronic. For acute gout systemic symptoms include fever and leukocytosis and increased inflammation while for chronic gout there is less inflammation but increased deformities of the bone. As part of the clinical features overtime there could be deposit of urates in internal organs. Other symptoms associated with arthritis generally include fatigue, fever, facial rash, headache, sleeping trouble, weight loss and major sites of arthritis are the knees, wrist, metatarsals, elbow, ankles and shoulders [1].

Arthritis and Diet

Although there is no diet cure for arthritis, certain foods have been shown to fight inflammation, strengthen bones and boost the immune system. Adding these foods to daily balanced diet may help ease the symptoms of arthritis and could help to prevent developing arthritis.

Anti-Inflammatory Diet for Arthritis

High fibre foods, fruits and vegetables, fish, nuts and beans, foods rich in antioxidants, diets low in processed foods and low saturated fat are important for lowering blood pressure, protecting against chronic conditions ranging from cancer to stroke, curbs inflammation, benefits hearts and joints, lead to desirable weight loss to manage joint pain. Adopting the 'Mediterranean diet' which consists of antioxidant rich foods such as poultry, fish, less lean red meat, wholegrain cereals, fresh fruit such as oranges, avocado, apples, cherries, plenty of vegetables (fresh, frozen or canned), olive oil, rapeseed oil, peas and beans and nuts and seeds is also a major way to stay healthy especially for those suffering from arthritis [1]. Olive oil is rich in oleic acid which has an anti-inflammatory effect similar to that of fish oil. For cases of juvenile rheumatoid arthritis which is associated with retarded growth and protein energy malnutrition as a result of articular inflammation and anaemia it is necessary to ensure that adequate nutrition is adopted to improve growth and development.

Fishes such as mackerel, tuna, salmon, snapper, sardine that are rich in omega 3 polyunsaturated fatty acid are recommended for people suffering from arthritis. These types of fish are good for the heart and their oils are beneficial for reducing inflammation at joints [7]. However, it is crucial not to confuse fish oils with fish liver oils (such as cod liver oil and halibut liver oil) because fish liver oils also contain vitamin A. and large amounts of vitamin A can cause serious side effects. Plant sources of Omega-3 fats include linseed, flaxseed and borage oil which could also be beneficial although not as much as the fish oil. Dietary modification for those who suffer from gout may include consuming a healthy diet by avoiding foods high in purines, including offal such as kidney, liver, seafoods such as herrings, sardines, shellfish such as prawns and they should avoid products containing yeast such as beer and most importantly they should drink plenty of water. They should also eat and drink moderately (no binge drinking/eating) and avoid rushing their meals. Foods high in trans fatty acid such as margarine and baked products should be consumed minimally [1].

Reduced levels of Omega 3 have resulted in problems such as hyperactivity, depression, numbness and tingling in the hands and feet and this are underlying causes of heart disease, asthma and auto-immune disease like rheumatoid arthritis. Western diet contains more omega 6 fatty acid than omega 3 fatty acid and an imbalance results in an inflammation. Maintaining balance in fatty acid plays an important role in inflammation control and its related health challenges. Evidences from scientific studies have shown that high levels of arachidonic acid, an omega-6 fatty acid is associated with people suffering with osteoarthritis. High levels of arachidonic acid result in an increased production of the pro-inflammatory eicosanoid hormones called prostaglandins, leukotrienes, and thromboxanes. Therefore, consumption of foods such as beef, eggs, organ meats and dairy products high in arachidonic acid could result in an inflammation however; reduction in their consumption will be of much dietary benefit [8].

Best sources of nuts include walnuts, peanuts, almonds etc. A recent study by the American Journal of Clinical nutrition (2011) found that amongst men and women that consumed nuts, there is a 51% lower risk of mortality due to an inflammatory disease compared to those who consumed lesser nuts while another study found that subjects with lower levels of vitamin B_6 which is found in most nuts had higher levels of inflammatory markers where there is no definitive arthritis diet. Vitamin B_6 functions in the metabolism of amino acids, it is essential for formation of red blood cells and metabolism and iron transport in the body. Foods rich in vitamin B_6 include whole grain foods, eggs, poultry, peanuts and dairy products. However, research suggests including anti-inflammatory foods in the diet and limiting foods that may trigger joint pain [6].

Three major amino acids are important in inflammation reduction. These are cysteine, glutathione, and taurine. Cysteine is an important amino acid for the production of the antioxidant glutathione. Glutathione plays major role in inflammatory response. Methionine is synthesized from homocysteine by Vitamin B_{12} in aminoacid metabolism and from folate in S-adenosylmethionine (SAMe) production which aids DNA synthesis and methylation.

S-adenosylmethionine has been proven to reduce degenerative damage and symptoms of osteoarthritis in patients, including related depression. It is necessary to consume foods rich in folate and vitamin B_{12} such as broccoli, spinach, eggs, meat and oranges. Thus those having gout might want to reduce folate intake because it synthesizes purines [8].

Another amino acid, glutamine responsible for glucosamine production is essential in diet because of its ability to produce cartilage tissues. Glucosamine aids the production of glycosaminoglycans, hyaluronic acid and proteoglycans. These substances form the basis of body tissues such as membranes of the respiratory and digestive system, tendons, ligaments, cartilage, collagen and synovial fluid in the joints. For instance, proteoglycans are proteins that make up the connective tissue of cartilage giving joints their elasticity, strength, and resilience. However, glucosamine supplements aid the production of elastic thick fluids which increases the joint support [6].

Consumption of iron rich foods such as vegetables, beans, eggs and peas is important for arthritis patients because the effect of inflammation on the body might be severe and this may lead to anaemic conditions. However to improve iron absorption in the body, foods rich in vitamin C should be consumed with the iron rich meal [7], for instance, eating fruits alongside with the meal or taking a glass of fruit juice with the meal. Iron deficiency anaemia may develop as a result of chronic inflammation resulting from poor dietary intake and gastrointestinal blood loss.

Calcium rich foods such as low fat milk, cheese, yoghurt and green leafy vegetables should be consumed. The bones require this calcium for growth, strength and movement and also to prevent osteoporosis [7].

Vitamins and minerals are beneficial in the management of arthritis. This is due to their antioxidant properties which are effective in defending and neutralizing reactive oxygen species (ROS) by enzymes such as superoxide dismutase, catalase and peroxidase. For instance in osteoarthritis where there is an increased production of ROS the antioxidant capacity of cells and tissues can become insufficient to detoxify the ROS, and this leads to cartilage degradation by inhibiting matrix synthesis and degrading matrix molecules. Vitamin C has a positive effect on reducing cartilage loss and osteoarthritis generally as proven from Framingham epidemiological study. Vitamin E has been shown to be beneficial to arthritis patients because of its anti-oxidant effect in preventing the activities of free radicals. Also foods rich in β-carotene will be of health benefit to arthritis patients because of its ability to quench singlet oxygen which may reduce the free radical burden and protect lipids from peroxidation [1]. Food sources from the nightshade group such as potatoes should be consumed minimally because the glucoalkaloid, solanine present in potatoes have the tendency to increase inflammation [2].

However, combining modest weight loss plus moderate exercise provides an improved body function in the performances measures of movement in older overweight and obese adults with knee osteoarthritis compared with either intervention methods carried out alone [9].

Also the introduction of enriching processed foods and beverages with specific non-encapsulated neutraceuticals (precisely anti-inflammatory agents from plants extracts) could significantly assist in preventing, managing and control inflammation of the joint that could have resulted into different forms of arthritis if left untreated. Fortunately there are wide ranges of plants and herbs that contain phenolic substances such as tannins, flavanol, flavonoids, anthocyanins, beta-carotene (which can be utilized for developing wide array of nutraceuticals that can be used to enrich foods and beverages such as mango, black pepper Indian ginseng, milkweed, aloe vera, ginger and turmeric/curcumin [10]. These compounds have been implicated to play significant role in scavenging for free radicals that are developed in normal physiological conditions of man due to oxidative stress. They possess anti-inflammatory properties, reducing properties and anti-oxidant properties. These anti-oxidant properties will play a great role in preventing lipid peroxidation and help to scavenge for free radicals such as hydroxyl free radical, nitric oxide free radical, DPPH free radical which if unchecked could bring about inflammation in the joint areas of the body [8, 11].

Physical therapy involving exercises could help to strengthen the muscles around the affected joint which is a core component of arthritis treatment. Weight loss and maintaining a healthy weight can reduce the symptoms in those that have osteoarthritis and they are also effective in reducing the risk of developing it.

Modification by Physical Activity

Regular physical activity with moderate vigour equally improves the quality of life and muscle function in patients suffering from RA however at the initial stage it could cause pain at the joints but after a continual process the pain becomes minimal. There are some suitable forms of exercise that patients suffering from RA can take part in, this include walking, dancing, light fitness, cycling, cross-country skiing, nordic walking, water gymnastics and strength training. Exercises involving muscle stretching and strengthening could be carried out by patients suffering from arthritis without causing them pain or stiffness. Children and teenagers should engage in about 60 minutes or more of physical activity each day [12]. During exercises or sports, it is essential that proper sporting kits are worn to prevent joint injury. Physical activity helps to reduce symptoms of stress, anxiety, depression and also stop social isolation. The positive effect of physical activity on patients suffering from RA have been associated with an alternation with the neuropeptide concentration and elevated serum concentration of IGF-1 [12].

Maintaining Normal Body Weight

Maintaining a healthy body weight is important in the prevention and management of arthritis. Overweight and obese people are susceptible to joint pain, swellings and stiffness. In order to minimize the possibly of suffering from arthritis healthy diet must be adopted and regular exercise must be done. Findings from the Framingham cohort studies indicates that weight loss of about 5 kg will reduce a person's risk of developing knee osteoarthritis over the subsequent 10 years by 50% [9].

Reduction of Fat in Diet

Patients suffering from arthritis should minimize the amount and type of fat consumed in their diets especially saturated fat. Oils containing high cholesterols should be reduced from their meals during cooking and consumption of fried foods should be minimized to prevent heart disease particularly those suffering from RA because of their higher heart disease risk. Using more of monounsaturated and polyunsaturated fat is beneficial for a healthy heart [7].

Management and Prevention

In managing arthritis it is important that before cutting down some certain meals from diet it is advisable to speak with a dietician or doctor (a rheumatologist) so that appropriate diagnose is known and beneficial meals are not overly restricted. Presently, no primary prevention has been determined for RA although, some studies showed smoking to be a risk factor however there is no modifiable risk factor to develop primary prevention mechanism for RA. In managing osteoarthritis the major target goal is to reduce pain and slow down the disease progression.

Heat and cold therapy could be adopted in arthritis management. The heat therapy involves taking a warm bath or using a towel soaked in warm water or a warm pack to massage or wrap around the inflamed joint for few minutes this method helps to reduce tightness and muscle spasm. It should be noted that in using a warm pack a towel could be placed around it to prevent direct heat contact to the inflamed joint so as not to aggravate the pain. The cold therapy involves the use of crushed ice cubes or blocks in a cold pack wrapped with a towel and placed on the joint, this method reduces swelling and pain [12].

Joints could be protected from strenuous activities by alternating activities with more stress with those of lesser stress, avoiding squatting, kneeling and uncomfortable positions, adopting a good and convenient sitting position and using helpful tools in carrying out duties for instance the use of carts to lift objects. Relaxing the muscles around inflamed joints is necessary to prevent pain and management of arthritis [12].

Clinical test such as ESR (erythrocyte sedimentation rate) which is a non-specific screening test for various diseases and C-reactive protein test which measures the concentration of protein in serum that indicates inflammation should be carried out to diagnose arthritis. However more specific tests such as fatty acid analysis, intestinal permeability assessment, comprehensive digestive stool analysis and amino acid test are required to determine the cause of the arthritis [2].

For secondary prevention, anti-inflammatory medications can be administered at the early stages provided symptoms are detected early. Therefore, adults should undergo early diagnosis and, on the onset of any symptom related to joint disorders or inflammations, frequent diagnosis and treatments should be carried out every 3 months. Homeopathy (this involves the use of herbs from plants or animals to induce healing abilities) has no proven scientific evidence but it does not constituent any harm either on the patient and massage could equally be given to arthritic patients to relieve them of the pain [2, 12].

TREATMENTS OF ARTHRITIS

Rheumatoid arthritis (RA) as well as the other forms of arthritis can be treated with medication, surgery and various forms of rehabilitation therapy. Some of the major medications given to patients suffering from rheumatoid arthritis include non-steroid anti-inflammatory drugs (NSAID), cortisone, slow acting anti-rheumatic drugs (SAARD) and disease-modifying anti-rheumatic drugs (DMARD) [12]. However, biological treatments such as TNF-alpha blockers and inhibitors, interleukin 1, CD 20+ B-cells and T-cells co-stimulation can also be administered. In order to prevent joint damages and disorders in the future inflammatory inhibitors should be given to patients who shows signs of RA early enough. Another effective anti-inflammatory medicine that can be administered into inflamed joint through injection or as a tablet is cortisone [2].

CONCLUSION

In arthritis prevention and management diets rich in fruits, vegetables, nuts and whole grains are advised alongside reduction of saturated fat, sugar and salt intake. Foods rich in antioxidant with anti-inflammatory effects are more beneficial in arthritis management, so also is weight management and increased physical activity.

REFERENCES

[1] O'conner A. Diet and Arthritis. British Nutrition Foundation; 2011. Available from: http://www.foodafactoflife.org.uk/attachments/dd125679-db74-4a9823ffdbc5.pdf.

[2] Grisanti RJ. How to Prevent and Treat Arthritis Pain with Nutritional Medicine. Ashland, Oregon: Sequoia Educational system; 2004.

[3] CDC Centres for Disease Control and Prevention. ARTHRITIS: Meeting the Challenges of Living well at a glance 2014. Atlanta: National Center for Chronic Disease Prevention and Health Promotion, 2014. Available from: http://www.cdc.gov/chronicdisease/resources/publications/aag/pdf/2014/arthritis-aag-2014.pdf.

[4] Prosser N, Webb M. Primary and secondary prevention of rheumatoid arthritis. Public Health Wales NHS Trust; 2010.

[5] Alam SM, Kidwai AA, Jafri SR, Qureshi BM, Sami A, Qureshi HH, et al. Epidemiology of Rheumatoid Arthritis in a tertiary care unit, Karachi, Pakistan. *J. Pak. Med. Assoc*. 2011; 61(2): 123-6.

[6] Medical Research Council (MRC). Diet and Arthritis - a report prepared by scientists at the Medical Research Council Human Nutrition Research at the request of The Arthritic Association; 2001. Available from: http://www.palindromicrheumatism.org/leaflet/Diet_and_Arthritis_.pdf.

[7] Schenker S. Diet and Rheumatoid Arthritis. Food Fact Sheet. The British Dietetic Association; 2015. Available from: https://www.bda.uk.com/foodfacts/Arthritis.pdf.

[8] Rennie KL, Hughes J, Lang R, Jebb SA. Nutritional management of rheumatoid arthritis: a review of the evidence. The British Dietetic Association Ltd. *J. Hum. Nutr. Dietet.* 2003; 16: 97–109.

[9] Pattison D. Diet and osteoarthritis. Food Fact Sheet. The British Dietetic Association; 2015. Available from: https://www.bda.uk.com/foodfacts/OsteoArthritis.pdf.

[10] Darlington LG, Stone TW. Antioxidants and fatty acids in the amelioration of rheumatoid arthritis and related disorders. *British J Nutr.* 2001; 85: 251-269.

[11] The Arthritic Society. Rheumatoid arthritis: Causes, Symptoms and Treatments; 2015. Available from: http://arthritis.ca/getmedia/6c39edce-5b2d-498d-bd60-28d33f3e1850/Rheumatoid-Arthritis-Causes-Symptoms-and-Treatments.pdf.

In: Diets and Diseases: Causes and Prevention
Editor: Wenbiao Wu
ISBN: 978-1-63484-580-9

Chapter 9

DIET: OVERWEIGHT AND OBESITY

Oluwatoyin Bolanle Oluwole*, Olubunmi Phebean Ibidapo, Temiloluwa Adebola Adesioye and Adebukola Adekemi Agboola
Department of Food Technology, Federal Institute of Industrial Research, Oshodi, Lagos, Nigeria

ABSTRACT

A detailed review about the association of diet with overweight and obesity is extensively discussed in this chapter. The causes and symptoms of overweight and obesity, diet-related treatment of overweight and obesity are discussed. Also, possible methods of reducing obesity and overweight are proposed at individual level, via research and development as well as through the food industries in form of consumption and production of healthy food products. Food and food products such as fruit and vegetables, high fibre meals, high fibre snacks, high fibre drinks, whole grain meals, etc. at predetermined levels of consumption should be encouraged globally. Several nutritional campaign or education against overweight and obesity needs to be conducted particularly in most developing countries in Africa where overweight and obesity is seen as an index of affluence and quality life.

Keywords: overweight, obesity, causes, diet, reduce, research, campaign, industries

INTRODUCTION

Obesity is defined as the disruption of energy balance or excess accumulation of body energy in form of fat that impairs health. It is an abnormal increase of body fat, usually about 20% or more over an individual ideal body weight. Obesity is associated with a higher risk of illness, impairment and mortality. Obesity is one of the major nutrition related disease of public health concern. Globally, overweight has become one of the factors of double burden

* Corresponding Author address: Department of Food Technology, Federal Institute of Industrial Research, Oshodi, Lagos, Nigeria. Email: oluwatoyinoluwole575@yahoo.com.

of malnutrition which needs to be addressed. Obesity can be classified according to the World Health Organization (WHO) [1] as Table 1.

Measures of obesity include:

- Body Mass Index (BMI) – It is a method widely used to measure obesity. It is calculated as the ratio of weight to height square.

$$\text{BMI} = \frac{\text{Weight (kg)}}{\text{Height}^2\,(\text{m}^2)}$$

However, BMI does not distinguish between the fat accumulations in the body whether it is in the lean tissue or in the abdomen.

- Absolute body fat
- Skin fold thickness
- Abdominal fat – useful index of shape and obesity associated with disease risk
  - – Waist hip ratio
  - – Waist circumference [2].

Table 1. Classification of Body Weight

Classification	BMI (kg/m^2)	Risk of comorbidities
Underweight	<18.5	Low (but risk of other clinical problems increased)
Normal range	18.5-24.9	Average
Overweight	>25	
Pre-obese	25.0-29.9	Increased
Obese class I	30.0-34.9	Moderate
Obese Class II	35.0-39.9	Severe
Obese Class III	>40.0	Very severe

The waist and hip circumference can give some useful data regarding risk factors associated with obesity. The higher the ratio, the greater the chance for weight- associated complications. Coronary disease, hypertension, type 2 diabetes mellitus, increased heart attack, hyperlipidemia, infertility and a higher preponderance of endometrial, colon, prostrate and breast cancer are severe health challenges related to people with excessive weight.

EPIDEMIOLOGY

Obesity in the World

According to the World Health Organization [3], in year 2014, more than 1.9 billion adults, 18 years and older were overweight, of these over 600 million were obese.

- Globally In year 2014, about 13% of the adult populations (11% of men and 15% of women) were obese while 39% of adults (38% of men and 40% of women) were overweight.
- Between 1980 and 2014, obesity prevalence has doubled worldwide.
- In year 2013, 42 million children under the age of five [5] were overweight and obese.
- However globally, about 170 million children (aged less than 18 years) are now estimated to be overweight.
- Currently, overweight and obesity kills more of the world's population than underweight.
- Obesity is preventable.

Obesity in Africa

According to a recent study it was observed that in Gambia, the male population had a lower overweight prevalence of about 10% compared to females in Sierra Leone with a 44% prevalence rate [4]. According to Abubakari et al. the average body mass index from twenty eight studies from a meta-analysis conducted on West Africa adult gave 20.1 to 27.0kg [5]. Therefore, obesity was more common amongst women than men with a prevalent rate of 10%. Those who reside in urban areas tend to be more obese than the rural dwellers as shown from results of a time trend analyses in West Africa, obesity prevalence doubled to about 114% in 15 years and this was common amongst women. Results from the first South African Demographic and Health Survey (SADHS) in Southern African sub-region, showed that more than 29% of men and 56% of women were overweight and obese [6]. This result shows that South Africa has a higher overweight and obesity prevalence than other African countries [7]. For both urban and rural women the issue of obesity is a serious challenge due to an increase in BMI with age. In addition, amongst the younger age groups (15-24 years) who are the adolescents and young people they are also at risk of this overweight and obesity epidemic. In spite of this, the double burden of malnutrition is also of significance in this sub-region. Another study conducted on low income elderly people in a South African community revealed that a higher number of the population are deficient in micronutrients such as zinc, they also had food security issues and majority of them were overweight and obese as well as hypertensive [8]. This shows the evidence of obesity, under nutrition in children as well as HIV/AIDS as a threatening disease in the South African population.

In the Northern sub-region, Belahsen and Rguibi [9] reported the results obtained from an obesity study carried out in six North African countries (Morocco, Mauritania, Algeria, Libya, Tunisia and Egypt). The results reported on obesity ranged from 13% to 46% in women, 4% to 22% in men, and 9% - 18% in school children and adolescents. However, obesity and its related diseases have become a significant health problem in these regions. In another study, Benajiba et al. [10] examined the similarities on obesity trends in Morocco and Spain. Their findings indicated similarity in the prevalence of obesity amongst adult in both countries (13%), in the last two decades however the prevalence doubled in Spain (Europe), but tripled in Morocco (Africa). Generally, there is a rise in figure in all African sub-regions.

Causes and Symptoms

The Mechanism of Excessive Weight Gain

Fat is stored in the adipose tissues as a result of excessive consumption of calories than the body can utilize. The precise cause of weight gain may arise from complex combination of factors. Genetic factors significantly determine the process involved in regulation of appetite in the body and the rate at which food is converted into energy (metabolic rate). However, a genetic trait or family history of gaining weight does not determine the possibly of one being obese. Another factor that can play a significant role in the amount of weight a person gain is the eating habit and patterns and forms of physical activity.

Recent studies have shown that the amount of fat present in a diet may have a greater effect on weight than the amount of calories it contains. Most fat calories are stored in fat cells and this gradually adds to the body's weight and girth as they expand and multiply.

A sedentary life style, which is particularly prevalent in affluent societies, can contribute to weight gain. Several other factors play a role in weight gain and one of such are psychological factors such as depression and low self-esteem which may in some cases influence one's eating habit. The ability to easily lose weight is however dependent on the stage of life when obesity sets in for an individual. Obesity can also be a side effect of certain disorders and conditions which includes cushing's syndrome, hypothyroidism, neurologic disturbance and the usage of drugs such as antidepressants, steroids and antipsychotic medications.

Obesity can give rise to several secondary conditions such as: arthritis, hyperlipidaemia, hypertension, abnormal glucose tolerance, infertility heartburn, high serum cholesterol levels, gall stones, high blood pressure, cardiovascular, atherosclerosis, menstrual irregularities or cessation of menstruation (amenorrhea), decreased fertility, pregnancy complications, asthma, lower back pain, hernias, gum disease, shortness of breath, sleep apnoea, skin disorders, emotional and social problems.

Becoming overweight or obese does not occur in a day but daily accumulation of unhealthy or excessive consumption of food increases its effect. Some people become overweight and eventually obese because of poor eating timing; such people eat high calorie or fatty food at night and sleep almost immediately without proper digestion of such meals. However, such constant habit causes excessive weight gain overtime.

Causes of Obesity

The major cause of obesity and overweight is when the amount of calories consumed is more than the amount of calories expended, thus, an energy imbalance occurs. Generally, in the world today it is on record that an increased consumption rate of energy dense foods that is high in fat and a decline in physical activities due to increased sedentary lifestyles as a result of work pattern, increased urban migrants and dwellers and varying transportation system all contribute to overweight and obesity.

Factors that contribute to obesity include: social, economic, genetic, psychological and environmental.

- Economic factors that influence the prevalence of obesity include poverty, the tendency for people to purchase more energy dense/fatty foods because of the quick satisfaction easily derived from their consumption and the low cost of purchasing such food items due to the low income earned.

  In the 21st Century, the poor prefer to consume foods which provide the most calories for the least money. With low purchasing power,as a result of limited budget, it is difficult for them to ensure consumption of diet rich in fruits and vegetables but low in fat and sugar. The priority of this category of people is to ensure that their household gets enough calories throughout the day. Unfortunately, foods that are particularly energy dense such as cakes, biscuits, candies and soft drinks are cheap per kcal compared to fruit and vegetables, meat and dairy foods. Overconsumption of energy dense foods rich in fat and sugar will gradually lead to obesity. The gradient in the economic cost of food in relation to energy density was nicely established in a French community study [11].

  Accessibility to food also influences the diet pattern of individuals, for instance people dwelling in places far from open markets, super markets may have difficulties getting the right meals because of the cost of transportation and distance involved in having to buy food stuffs. This situation may influence their food uptake generally and more especially their eating pattern.

  The affluent are also at greater risk of obesity because of their quick access to purchase food especially unhealthy ones while eating out and the comfort they derive while seated in a vehicle driven by a driver all day hereby neglecting the need to undergo any form of exercise especially, if it is a door to door driven service. The use of elevators at all times instead of the stairs can also result in poor activity levels.
- Genetic factor which influences obesity includes leptin deficiency (leptin is a receptor located in the adipocytes that control appetite regulation therefore reducing the urge to eat and increasing energy expenditure) and other hereditary factors [12]. However, research evidence has proved that leptin deficiency is very rare in human this implies that obese people are not deficient in leptin rather other factors are responsible for their obese nature. Obesity could also be hereditary especially in families with previous records of obesity. Also several monogenic factors can cause human obesity such as the Prader-willi, Bardet-Biedl and Klinefelter syndromes.
- Psychological factors are being influenced by the advertising media, for instance children are more captivated by the food adverts made on the media and will long for such meals whether such products are healthy or not. Also peer group influence might affect eating pattern of children and this may allow them to eat more than usual particularly when they are in groups or in company of other colleagues than while eating alone [13]. Increase in food consumption can be influenced by the pleasure or love for such meals and this causes increasing weight overtime.
- Environmental and cultural factors that have an effect on obesity include weight gained after marriage due to increased parity and the possibility of gaining more weight with increasing age. However, social class gradient has associated individuals with large protruding bellies as a sign of good living and affluence whereas in the main sense such individuals have increased abdominal waist circumference which is detrimental to their health.

- **Social Factors - dietary factors and physical activity:** Social factors that are underlying causes of obesity include: high calorific diet intake, the portion size of food and the type of food consumed have a great impact in contributing to obesity. Foods high in saturated fat, high cholesterol and poor nutritive meals all contribute towards obesity. Another social factor is lack or inadequate physical activity and sedentary lifestyle especially for those who often play computer games and watch television for long hours. There is a tendency for them to eat more food on the same spot without any involvement in bodily exercise [14]. Usually, when energy expenditure is lesser than energy intake in a person who is susceptible to weight gain, then obesity sets in [15, 16]. Measuring energy intake and expenditure is difficult and different methods have been used in various studies. This may explain partly the inconsistent relationship between these factors and obesity. Food intake has been associated with obesity not only in terms of the volume of food ingested but also in terms of the composition and quality of diet. Furthermore, there has been a shift in eating habits over time. Presently, there is a tendency for children to avoid eating breakfast, consume less fruits and vegetables but they would rather consume more drinks, snacks and sweets and all these products increase their chances of becoming obese over time [17]. In a review by Moreno and Rodriguez [16], it was concluded that well breastfed infants had a lesser risk of becoming obese while those that consume high energy meals and sugar based beverages were at risk of becoming obese even as a child and later in life when they become adults [18, 19]. With regards to other dietary habits, Nicole et al. [20] found an association between dieting and skipping meals with a risk of 3.98 (95% CI: 1.83-8.67) and 2.54 (95% CI: 1.22- 5.29) respectively. Also, there was a higher incidence rate of obesity in adolescents who ate meals outside the home [21].

Other causes of overweight and obesity could include the effect of having to sit long hours in traffic daily as common in places like Lagos, Nigeria and individuals are left with the option of compulsorily buying snacks and fizzy drinks. Overtime unconsciously the desire to consume healthy meals at home is limited due to fatigue and this fast meal replaces the good healthy meal which should have been consumed.

Common Health Consequences of Overweight and Obesity

- Cardiovascular diseases (Mainly heart disease and stroke) which were the leading cause of death in year 2012.
- Diabetes
- Musculoskeletal disorders such as osteoarthritis- a highly disabling degenerative disease of the joints.
- Some cancers (endometrial, breast and colon).

Childhood obesity is associated with a higher chance of obesity, premature death and disability in adulthood. Also obese children experience breathing difficulties, increased risk of fractures, hypertension, early markers of cardiovascular disease, insulin resistance and psychological effects.

Control of Obesity

Controlling obesity requires a gradual process which includes: taking part in physical activities, using more of the stairs than elevators, reducing calorie and fat intake, reducing alcohol consumption, reducing the intake of fizzy drinks, candies etc, increasing the consumption of fruits and vegetables and increasing fibre intake [22].

At the individual level, people can limit energy intake from fats and sugars, increase consumption of fruits and vegetables as well as legumes, whole grains and nuts, and engage in regular physical activity (60 minutes per day for children and 150 minutes per week for adults).

The Food Industry

The food industry can play a significant role in promoting healthy diets by:

1. *Reducing the fat, sugar and salt content of processed foods.*

   Processed foods are foods with alterations from their natural state either for convenience, safety or preservation. Examples of commonly processed foods may include, cheese, soft drinks, milk, crisps, bacon, tinned vegetables and breakfast cereals. Processed foods themselves might not be always unhealthy but the addition of sugar, salt and fat for flavor enhancement, as a part of the food structure as in the case of cakes and bread and to extend their shelf life may have adverse effect if not done minimally.

   Food industries should ensure that there is minimal addition of sugar and salt to food during processing. For instance, in salted popcorn, caution should be made during addition of salt to handy snacks like this especially for individuals who might not be aware of their health challenges on time. Addition of sugar to juice should be minimal, instead natural juice with its natural sugars should be encouraged, however if it should be further sweetened the quantity of sugar added must be considered. Furthermore, some processed foods like meats have high fat content such as bacon, salami, sausages and ham. It is therefore important that proper labeling preferably using colour coding styles and packaging is done to inform the buyer of the health implication of consuming large portion sizes of such foods daily.
2. *Ensuring that healthy and nutritious choices are available and affordable to all consumers.*

   Skimmed milk, low fat milk and yoghurts should be made affordable for all classes of people to break the barrier of low and high class consumption of nutritious meals.

3. *Practicing responsible marketing strategies especially those aimed at children and teenagers.*

   Children and teens are fast learners and hence they adapt well to their environments. Food industries should imbibe attractive marketing strategies with clear details of nutritious and healthy food products.
4. *Ensuring the availability of healthy food choices and supporting regular physical activity in the workplace.*

   As part of Corporate Social Responsibilities (CSR), food industries could organize sporting activities weekly, fortnightly, monthly or quarterly in communities, schools, organizations and even as social activities amongst their staffs promoting the need for regular exercise. Alongside, they could advertise the importance of consuming their products and give control on portion sizes if such meals have high calories or fat.

However, in trying to reduce significantly the population of overweight and obese individuals, high calorie and fatty foods should not be administered to people in the same manner as drugs are being prescribed to patients, as it is difficult to control people's eating pattern except they are under close surveillance. On the other hand, a particular food product may not provide the required recommended daily allowance for fat intake however, inadequate knowledge on consumption of high fatty foods may expose people to uncontrollable consumption of those products. Parents and guardians should hereby assist to monitor the eating pattern of their children to prevent them from becoming obese progressively, by cutting down overconsumption of foods high in calories, fat and sugar.

Other ways of controlling obesity include carrying out surgery on obese patients; such operations include the gastric bypass method, gastric banding and the vertical banding gastroplasty (VBG).

Prevention of Obesity

Strategies to be carried out in preventing obesity includes campaign on educating people on nutritional labels on food products, sign posts showing nutritional tips on weight loss and eating healthy, encouraging physical activities among individuals, in schools and local communities, improving the income of the populace which will enable them spend more on purchasing healthy meals, encourage breastfeeding and reducing fat and calorie intake [14].

There is an urgent need for government, non-governmental organizations, National Nutritional societies, Food science and technology societies, Medical societies, Public health experts to come together through a stakeholders meeting and strategize as to the best methods of embarking on nutritional campaign against overweight and obesity with provision of adequate information on their prevention, management and control to the populace at all levels of governance (local, states and federal levels). This proposed nutritional campaign could be done via the media, radio, television and through seminars organized at local, states and federal levels interpreted into different local languages for maximum comprehension to be able to get to the grassroot populace and the general public as much as possible.

Also organizations in charge of regulating the quality of food products in the country as well as those setting standards for processed food products should be checked to promote and monitor the production of healthy processed food products for the citizenry.

The government should also make policies that will influence the food environment which are likely to be effective interventions that include restrictions on the marketing of unhealthy foods. The food sector should be monitored and checked against processing of unhealthy food for the populace, strategies on sensitizing people on the importance of nutrition labeling should be carried out. In addition to that, food manufacturers should include nutritional labels correctly and indicate those with high salt, sugar and fat so that everyone can have a quick understanding of what their food constitute. Food taxes and subsidies on healthy foods should be lesser so that everyone including the low income earners can afford eating healthy.

However, there are policies that influences conducive environment for physical activity which can be made effective through reducing barriers to physical activity, enacting laws on transport policies which will enhance a safe environment for those carrying out physical activities within the community especially along the walk ways, policies on space increment for recreational activities, and school-based physical activity policies should be implemented by ensuring all schools have field space or playing ground for students to carry out physical activities through integrating it in the school curriculum.

Another way to prevent overweight and obesity is through the use of food diaries. The food diary method helps individuals to take note of all the meals they consume per day and keep record of the portion sizes. Therefore a weighing balance is required to take the weight of all meals consumed at every point in time of the day for a specific period of time. Thereafter, the records are inputted into software that decodes the amount of energy, protein, fat and other necessary food parameters present in the consumed meal. Using this method enlightens and helps individual to know where they need to cut down certain food to maintain a healthy life. However, certain challenges are associated with this method, firstly there could be bias, individuals might not be consistent, truthful and honest in carrying it out daily and finally, there could be mistakes or inaccuracies. Despite all the challenges, this method is still a very good one for people willing to monitor their diet. The psychological aspect of this method is that individuals might be lazy to eat more because of the stress involved in weighing and keeping records. On the other hand, it could make them eat heavily all at once to minimize the effort required to weigh all other meals to be consumed.

Diet Related Treatment of Obesity

The type and quantity of food consumed – In order to monitor the quantity of food consumed and the nutritional composition, it is important that methods such as the use of the food diary, food frequency questionnaire can be adopted. However, the rate of food consumed can be affected by the timing and the rate of metabolism rate.

The mechanism that controls response to food – Appetite is regulated by several mechanism therefore some psychological factors may affect the body's response to food and this differs for each individual.

Modification by Exercise

Regular physical activity or exercise is an integral part of everyday life and this is key in achieving and maintaining weight loss. For most individuals who are mildly obese, this behavior modification requires adapting a different lifestyle which can be strictly abided by independently or being supervised by a family physician. Other mildly obese persons may seek the help of a commercial weight loss program which they can adopt and follow solely. For individuals who are moderately obese, there is a need to medically supervise their behavior changes in acquiring weight loss. A moderately obese person could require consuming a low calorie diet while some other individuals may require an extremely low calorie protein diet. For individuals who are severely obese, dietary changes and behavior modification may be accompanied by surgery to reduce/bypass portions of the stomach or small intestine. However, drugs that help in appetite suppression could also be prescribed to aid weight loss in obese people.

Anti-obesity drugs such as orlistat can be administered to obese patients with BMI of >30. This drug is given to those within the age 18-75 years. Prior to the administration of anti-obesity drugs certain examinations should be carried out, such as the BMI, blood pressure and waist circumference while investigations should be carried out on the fasting blood glucose, lipid profile and urinalysis.

Current Research and Development of Overweight and Obesity Prevention and Management

Developed value added product such as whole grain based extruded snacks and meals, high fibre meals, foods rich in antioxidants, nutraceuticals, low fat biscuits, low sodium, low sugar and fat meals and drinks, dried fruit snacks and vegetables at regulated levels of consumption depending on the initial body mass index, frequency of eating, psychological factors, genetic factors should be taken into consideration as well as the age of the target person involved before appropriate diet pattern can be recommended.

Interestingly, some of these value added healthy food products have been extensively worked on as research and development projects in the Department of Food Technology of the Federal Institute of Industrial Research, Oshodi, Lagos, Nigeria awaiting pilot plant production trials, clinical trials and eventual commercialization of the developed technologies. The use of enriching food and beverages with nanoencapsulated specific nutraceutical compounds could also help in reducing the incidence of development of other chronic disease such as diabetes and cardiovascular diseases in the populace who are already overweight/obese.

Conclusion

Obesity is majorly affected by unhealthy diets. Calories and fats are important in the body but an imbalance in energy accumulation and expenditure is a major factor that results in overweight and obesity. Individuals, governments and food industries have different roles to play in making sure that there is a reduction in mortality rates which emanates from overweight, obesity and their related health impairment.

REFERENCES

[1] WHO. Obesity: preventing and managing a global epidemic. WHO technical report series 894. WHO: Geneva; 2000.

[2] Geissler C, Powers H. Human nutrition. 12th ed. UK: Elsevier Limited; 2011.

[3] WHO Obesity and Overweight. Facts Sheet No 311; 2015. Available from: http://www.who.int/mediacentre/factsheets/fs311/en/(Last Accessed: 18th August, 2015).

[4] WHO. Global Info Base; 2006. Available from: www.who.int/ncd_surveillance/infobase/web.

[5] Abubakari AR, Bhopal RS. Systematic review on the prevalence of diabetes, overweight/obesity and physical inactivity in Ghanaians and Nigerians. *Pub Health.* 2008; 122(2): 173-182.

[6] Puoane T, Steyn K, Bradshaw D, Laubscher R, Fourie J, Lambert V, et al. (2002). Obesity in South Africa: the South African demographic and health survey. *Obes Res.* 2002; 10(10): 1038-1048.

[7] Goedecke JH, Jennings CL, Lambert EV. Obesity in South Africa. In: Steyn K, Fourie J, Temple N, editors. Chronic Diseases of Lifestyle in South Africa: 1995-2005. Medical Research Council – Technical Report. Tygerberg, W Cape: MRC; 2006. p. 65-79.

[8] Oldewage-Theron WH, Samuel FO. The Double Burden of Disease in African Elderly Attending a Care Centre in Sharpeville, South Africa. 1st Meeting of the Federation of the African Nutrition Societies (FANUS), Ouarzazate (Morocco), May 7-9 Africa. In: Steyn K, Fourie J, Temple N, editors. Chronic Diseases of Lifestyle in Africa 1995-2005, Technical Report. Cape Town: South Africa Medical Research Council; 2007.

[9] Belahsen R, Rguibi M. Obesity and Mediterranean Diet in North Africa. 1st Meeting of the Federation of the African Nutrition Societies (FANUS), Ouarzazate (Morocco), May 7-9, 2007.

[10] Benajiba N, Warnberg J, Aguenaou H, Marcos A. Obesity Prevalence and Trends: Comparison between Morocco and Spain. 1st Meeting of the Federation of the African Nutrition Societies (FANUS), Ouarzazate (Morocco), May 7-9, 2007.

[11] Darmon N, Briend A, Drewnowski A. Energy-dense diets are associated with lower diet costs: a community study of French adults. *Pub Health Nutr.* 2003; 7(1): 21-27).

[12] Speakman JR. Obesity: part two- The biology of body weight regulation. *Biologist* 2003; 50(2): 69-74.

[13] Speakman JR. Obesity: part one-the greatest health threat facing mankind. *Biologist* 2003; 50(1): 10-4.

[14] Dehghan M, Akhtar-Danesh N, Merchant AT. Childhood obesity, prevalence and prevention. *Nutr J.* 2005; 4: 24.

[15] Rosebaum M, Leibel RL, Hirsch J. Obesity. *N Engl J Med.* 1997; 337: 396-407.

[16] Moreno LA, Rodriguez G. Dietary risk factors for development of childhood obesity. *Curr Opin Clin Nutr Metab* Care. 2007; 10: (3) 336-341.

[17] Harley AJG, Harris SB, Gittelsohn J, Wolver TMS, Saksvig B, Zinman B. Overweight among children and adolescents in a native Canadian community: prevalence and associated factors. *Am J Clin Nutr*. 2000; 71: 693-700.

[18] Owen N, Leslie E, Salmon J, Fotheringham MJ. Environmental determinants of physical activity and sedentary behavior. *Exerc Sport Sci Rev*. 2000; 28(4): 153-158.

[19] Forshee RA, Anderson PA, Storey ML. Sugar-sweetened beverages and body mass index in children and adolescents: a meta-analysis. *Am J Clin Nutr*. 2008; 87(6): 1662-1671.

[20] Nicole GT, Ricardo TP, Bernardo LH, Karen ATP, Lucia LH. Prevalence and factors associated to overweight and obesity in adolescents. *Rev Saude Publica*. 2006; 40(4). http://dx.doi.org/10.1590/S0034-89102006000500011.

[21] Aggarwal T, Bhatia RC, Singh D, Sobti PC. Prevalence of obesity and overweight in affluent adolescents from Ludhiana, Punjab. *Indian Pediatr*. 2008; 45(6): 500-502.

[22] Swinburn BA, Caterson I, Seidell JC, James WPT. Diet, nutrition and the prevention of excess weight gain and obesity. *Pub Health Nutr*. 2004; 7(1A): 123–146.

In: Diets and Diseases: Causes and Prevention
Editor: Wenbiao Wu

ISBN: 978-1-63484-580-9

Chapter 10

OBESITY AND NUTRITION

Gulcin Algan Ozkok*

Vocational School of Health Sciences Child Development Program,
Selcuk University, Konya, Turkey

ABSTRACT

When people eat healthily, they feel healthy and work better, they have an increased performance at work, and they become happy as they feel socially well. Human body requires foods consumed externally in order to function properly. If we take more than enough calorie or the body doesn't burn enough calorie, body starts to store the extra energy. Today, fast-food products which are consumed largely by children or young people can cause lack of nutrition or malnutrition and therefore, they increase the risk of obesity. Obesity defined as the excessive fat tissue in the body, which affects over 300 million people according to the data of World Health Organization (WHO). Obesity spreads like an epidemic and it also becomes an economical burden by increasing health expenses of the countries. Nearly a billion people are obese.

Obesity is a serious health problem which causes various disorders through effecting mainly cardiovascular and endocrine system and it can even cause death. There are many factors effecting the development of obesity. Demographic factors, genetic susceptibility, environmental factors, behavioral factors, diet, eating habits and psychological factors are the most significant reasons of obesity. In the present study, these causes of obesity will be handled and behavioral factors, diet and eating habits will be examined in detail. In obesity disorder developed by wrong or unbalanced eating habits fat cell formation is very fast especially in the first few years of the life. The number of fat cells increases when fat storage becomes faster in the body. The number of fat cells for the obese children is three times more than normal weight children. Obese children diet indicates that they take extra energy from the fat. Eating style in babyhood determines the eating habits of a child later in life. Eating fast and chewing less are among the factors easing the development of obesity.

* Corresponding Author Address: Vocational School of Health Sciences Child Development Program, Selcuk University, Konya, Turkey. Email: gulcinalgan@selcuk.edu.tr.

Efforts to avoid obesity are the essence of fighting against this disease. In this respect, what is important is not to cure obesity well but to avoid it. Thus, starting from the fetal period, proper eating habits should be developed.

Keywords: obesity, nutrition, eating habits

INTRODUCTION

Nutrition provides the necessary food nutrients and energy for the body to ensure its continuation of vital activities, growth and development and to protect health continuously and in a balanced way. Eating food merely for pleasure or just to fill the stomach is not nutrition.

Ibn Sina, the nineteenth century Turkish philosopher, explained during his time how gluttony or eating for pleasure damages one's body and gave advice about the topic of nutrition according to his scientific findings which continue to apply even today. As well, Hippocrates and Celcus also reported before the twentieth century that some nutrients were not good for health and some others were necessary for health and people should be fed according to a certain scheme. Changes in social, economic or cultural life also affects eating habits over time. Becoming rich often causes an increase in the consumption of low nutritional foods that are refined instead of simpler, conventional foods [1]. At the present time, the number of those who migrate from villages to cities is increasing. When the state of families in the village changes from consuming what they produce to buying, they start to buy more sugary and starchy foods as they do not know the lack of value of the food they are buying [2]. In parallel with this change in the diet, the consumption of foods with high calories and less nutritional values is having an extreme effect on the length of life and health adversely. In cases of not eating properly, there will be changes in metabolic rate and as a result of unhealthy conditions the individual will start gaining fat. Obesity rates in the world are increasing every day, and while consumption is increasing, people's activity levels are decreasing during the day.

Obesity is widely regarded as the most important public health problem in the global dimension of the 21st century and is considered to be an increasing problem of coming in the coming years with the predominance of poor eating habits and the sedentary lifestyle of modern life.

The present study addresses the basic dimensions and measures to be taken against obesity, as well as determining the factors influencing obesity in order to develop recommendations for prevention. The sources related to the subject have been studied using the literature review technique.

OBESITY

Definition of Obesity

Obesity is the state of an excessive increase in body fat mass in proportion to non-fat mass and exceeding the expected body weight size compared to the height. According to

WHO's definition, obesity is the accumulation of fatty tissue disrupting the person's health [3].

It is known that obesity is a state of fat accumulation in the body attained from excessive consumption of foods. Obesus, is a Latin word which means because of eating [4]. In the past, obesity was a marker of high status and material wealth and was perceived as the physical appearance of a healthy person. While obesity was sometimes correlated to strength, power, sovereignty, imposing presence, fertility and abundance as a positive concept in the historical process, perceptions began to shift to refer to negative concepts such as lumpishness, trouble, being slow and unhealthy along with the industrial revolution [5]. Today, obesity is perceived as a harbinger of many systemic diseases. In the studies conducted, it is revealed that obesity was certainly a very important risk factor for diseases such as coronary heart disease, hypertension, stroke, type 2 diabetes, ovarian, breast, prostate and colon cancer, osteoarthritis (arthritis), varicose veins, sleep apnea syndrome, birth difficulties, ovarian cysts, and depression [6].

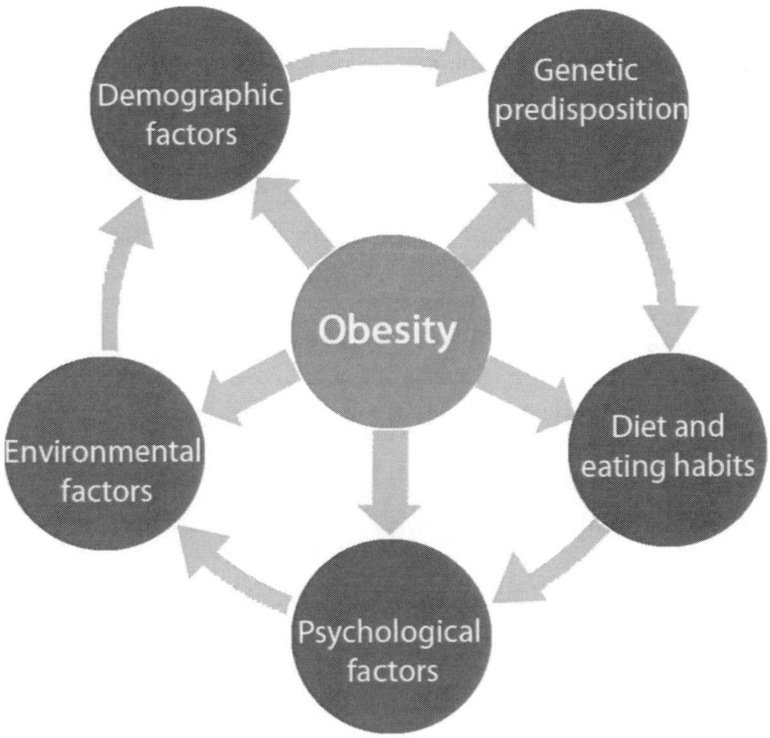

Figure 1. Factors that influence the formation of obesity.

Causes of Obesity

There are many factors affecting the formation of obesity, mainly; demographic factors, genetic predisposition, environmental factors, diet and eating habits and psychological factors. Factors that influence the formation of obesity are schematically depicted in Figure 1.

Demographic Factors

Age

Obesity is seen in every age but especially in recent years it seems to increase with age. The fat rate in the body increases with age. Obesity is not only seen in adult females or males but also in young children. It shows an increase in females and males depending on age, at least up to ages of 50 – 60 [7]. Obesity seen in childhood can possibly continue in every period of life when no prevention is taken [8]. Since 1999 the studies of "National Health and Nutrition Examination Survey (NHANES)" have been conducted in the United States considering Lowest and Most weight rates. The last research was conducted in 2012. The percentage of the prevalence of obesity in children under 2 years was determined as 8.1% and in 2-19 years old children it was found as 16.9% [9]. The World Health Organization (WHO) Regional Office for Europe reported that more than about 20% of children and adolescents in the European Region are overweight and one third of these children and adolescents are obese [10]. Obese children are likely to be obese in adulthood at a rate of twice as much more than normal weight children [11]. While the rate of overweight children was 15% and the rate of obese children was 5% in the United Kingdom in 1989, this ratio increased up to 24% and 9% in 1998 [12]. The detected prevalence obesity in adolescents between the ages 12-17 is still 8-25% in the whole of Europe. Obesity rates of some countries are as follows: Latin America (4.4%), Africa (3.9%) and Asia (2.9%) [13]. With a 10% rate, Russia had the lowest, and with 36% rate, Italy had the highest obesity rate among the countries reported [14].

Gender

The increase of estrogen during puberty in young people causes an increase of fat in body. With the influence of estrogen the fat begins accumulating in the body during adolescence and this is reflected as weight more in girls as the level of estrogen in girls is higher than it is in boys. Thus, obesity is higher among girls compared to boys during puberty. Akıs (2003) conducted a study in Bursa-Orhangazi with 5795 children who were 6-14 age group and found that the prevalence of obesity was more in girls than it was in boys [15]. Suzek (2005) conducted a study in Muğla with 6480 students who were between the ages of 6-15 and found that obesity prevalence was 7.6% for girls and 9.1% for boys. The findings also showed a high prevalence of obesity in age 10 [16]. It is known that the cause of weight increase in women is because of the pregnancy and birth processes. In addition, a number of biological conditions in which they experience during menopause can be the source of their weight problem [17].

Genetic Predisposition

Some of the factors causing obesity are genetic factors that are showing susceptibility to obesity and some others are environmental that are effecting later in life. Although there are not enough genetic studies in childhood, genetic factors are implicated in 40-70% of obesity in adults [18]. A single gene defect that could lead to obesity has been found in genetic studies [19, 20]. Ob gene located in leptin production and cocaine regulated by leptin and transcript (CART) protein regulated with amphetamine has drawn attention in recent years [21]. Studies on genes activating mechanisms other than leptin are also being conducted [22, 23].

In a cohort study involving three-generations in order to examine the genetic components of childhood obesity, it is stated that children's birth weight, eating habits and their weight in 3-5 years were noted as having similar features throughout three generations [24]. According to a systematic analysis examining the relationship between parents' BMI values and obesity in children, it has been indicated that particularly the maternal weight in pre-pregnancy may be related to the childhood obesity but studies on this subject are still not sufficient [25]. On the other hand, though it is suggested that there are genes increasing obesity predisposition in exogenous obesity, lifestyle and familial factors still carry more importance. In surveys conducted on families at risk, obesity probability in children with normal weight parents was found as 7%, whereas this probability was 40% with one obese parent and it increases to 80% when both parents were obese [26].

Environmental Factors

Sedentary lifestyle and eating foods that are high in calories and fat, as well as easy access to these foods, have become a common problem for not only developing countries but also developed countries in terms of environmental factors [27]. One of the most important factors regarding obesity is the imbalance of the amount of energy that is received and spent (not spending as much energy as it is received). The rapid increase in obesity prevalence in recent years all around the world has been linked to lifestyle changes. Nutrition habits shifting to lower quality foods and beverages containing less nutrients but more energy increase the amount of caloric intake. Besides, the limited number of places that children can play and do sports affects their amount of energy spent outside and causes them to spend long periods of time watching television or being on computer and lessens their energy expenditure [28]. It is known that watching television for long hours also has effects on preferring unhealthy foods and on habits of autonomic eating [29]. Having snacks and eating food containing with high fat, sugar and salt while watching TV also increase the imbalance between energy intake and energy expenditure. Inactivity is observed as a cause of obesity and obesity leads to lack of movement which constitutes a vicious circle. In a study conducted in the United States with 25% of overweight or obese children, sedentary habits such as watching television and using the computer have been identified as important factors in the development of obesity. Although there are no researches examining the relationship between computer use and obesity, there are studies showing that the excessive television watching (average of five hours or more daily) causes obesity in children. It is reported that as the amount of time that children spend on a computer increases (in addition to time spent watching television) the risk of obesity increases as well [30]. Weekly screen time for children is as high as 55 hours/week, and the average home in the United States has a television on for 8 hours per day [31, 32].

According to a systematic analysis examining the relationship between sleep duration and obesity, short sleep duration is mainly reported as an independent risk factor in the formation of obesity seen in children [33].

Diet and Eating Habits

Mother's nutrition during gestation can have a strong effect on future nutritional habits of the baby. Taste development primarily begins in utero [34]. In fetal exposure, fetus learns to accept and prefer the foods consumed by the mother. Amniotic fluid is renewed in every three hours. In last trimester, a fetus swallows an average of 1 lt amniotic fluid. Studies have indicated that foods consumed by the mother in last few hours of gestation change the taste of amniotic fluid. Moreover a fetus both smells and swallows the amniotic fluid during last months of gestation [35, 36]. As both amniotic fluid and breast milk include nutrient molecules from mother's diet, learning about taste of foods begins in utero and early fetal period [37].

The diversity, frequency, quantity and content of the diet administered from birth comprise the most important factors of children's eating habits. Starting to feed the child with energy-rich foods at an early age and giving these kinds of foods for long periods of time are practices that cause obesity and increase the child's stomach capacity. The preventive effect of breastfeeding on obesity formation is very well known. Adverse changes in the diet are also caused by the following factors: the increase in eating out and the consumption of sugar-sweetened beverages, an increase in portion size, the lack of nutritional diversity, eating fast food and snacks that are high in energy and fat which are quickly and easily accessible, as well as seemingly omnipresent [38, 39].

The effective factor for obesity is excessive eating habits. The speed of formation of new fat cells is particularly high earlier in life. As the fat accumulation accelerates, the number of fat cells also increases. The number of fat cells in obese children is approximately three times more than in normal children. Today, common factors which can cause obesity are: nutrition with extremely high calories, physical activity restriction, not having breakfast, and eating fast food high in sugar and calories.

Psychological Factors

There are many biological, psychological, social, and environmental factors involved in the etiology of obesity. Therefore, in the management of obese individuals, a multidimensional approach with psychological support is needed [40]. In both national and international studies, it is reported that people who are applying for the treatment of obesity are in need of a psychosocial support [41].

Mental and social problems such as lack self-confidence, negative body image, depression, suicide, smoking, alcohol and drug use, unemployment, loneliness, social exclusion and discrimination are seen in people who are obese. In obesity management, it is important to take into account body perception. Body dissatisfaction in obese individuals is associated with perceived body weight rather than actual body weight [42]. In a study it is found that self-esteem of overweight/obese people is lower than those with normal weight and the self-esteem value of obese people has a certain correlation with BMI (as BMI increases, self-esteem is found to be reduced). In another study it is found that there is a strong correlation between BMI and body dissatisfaction. Additionally, body image has strong effect on psychosocial health [43]. It is observed that psychopathological conditions accompanied by depression and personality disorders are more in obese patients [44]. It is reported that eating manner change of most people relates to emotional states such as being joyful, sad, stressed, etc. As a reaction to psychological problems, extreme anorexia can be seen in some children, while in others they can react by eating more. The relationship between parents and children, problems in the home environment, not being accepted by friends, and failure at school can affect individual's spiritual structure and cause malnutrition [45, 46].

Health Problems That Leads to Obesity

Obesity is globally a major public health problem. Obesity is considered to be one of the biggest health problems in the world. Obesity affects the health of the individual in various ways; it is difficult to move a heavy body. The disorders of various organs may lead to reduction in lifespan. The negative effects of obesity on human health are revealed by various studies. It is found that people who are between 40-44 years and 20% fatter have higher mortality rate (30-40% higher) than those with normal weight. But the rate in 40% of people of the same age with more weight increases up to 80-100% [47]. Some of the health problems caused by obesity are listed below.

Diabetes Mellitus

Diabetes mellitus is among the most important cardiovascular risk factors. Unfortunately, the incidence of diabetes is increasing rapidly in developed and developing countries. The most important causes of the increase in diabetes rate are the increase in overweight and obesity, sedentary lifestyle and the aging of the population. It is known that the increase in Type 2 diabetes rate is parallel with the increase in obesity. Among a number of risk factors, obesity and ethnicity are in the front row. BMI is found over 40 in one third of the adolescents with Type 2 diabetes, while in 17% of the adolescents BMI is found over 45 [48-49]. Type 2 diabetes prevalence is significantly higher in Africans, Mexicans and Native Americans. Another risk factor is gender: the male/female ratio is found as 1.7/1 [50, 51].

Metabolic Syndrome

Metabolic syndrome, which is an epidemic of our era, is a sickness increasing the risk of occurrence of cardiovascular disease- the most important disease causing death in our country and all over the world [52-54]. Metabolic syndrome is a disorder of the glucose and insulin balance resulting in an increase in blood fat in the body [55-57].

Hypertension

One of the most important diseases associated with obesity is hypertension. All over the world, especially in industrialized countries, obesity and hypertension are rapidly increasing. From at least 1/3 to 2/3 of hypertensive patients are obese. Hypertension is observed 3 times more in obese people [58, 59]. Framingham study also reports that more than 70% of hypertensive men and more than 60% of hypertensive women are obese. According to the results of the same study, when the weight is 20% above the ideal weight, the hypertension risk increases 8 times more [60, 61].

Cancer Types

In recent years, in parallel with the increasing of obesity incidence cancer and cancer types also increased. Especially in the West obesity is increasingly recognized as having a strong effect in the development of many types of cancer. It is reported that obesity increases the risk of some cancer types such as colon, rectum, esophagus, pancreas, breast and endometrium [62, 63]. Two thirds of adults in the US are increasingly overweight or obese. It is found that newly diagnosed cancer has been found to be associated with increased BMI in approximately 3.2% of men and in 8.8% of women [64].

Respiratory (Pulmonary) System Disorders

Obesity is a serious complication of Sleep Apnea Syndrome affecting respiratory system. Excess fat accumulation in the abdomen and chest wall can restrict breathing movements of the chest. For the morbidly obese the oxygen consumption required in respiratory processes is 3 times faster compared to the ones who are not obese [65]. Obesity is found approximately in 70-80% of individuals with sleep apnea. Studies conducted have shown that 10% increase in the body mass index increases the risk of sleep apnea 6% [66].

EVALUATION PROCEDURES FOR OBESITY

The most practical review of obesity is weight percent based on height. Weight-for-height is the ideal weight being between 90% -110%. If the weight is between 110-120% it is overweight, if it is above 120% it is obesity and if it is over 140% it is defined as morbid obesity [67]. Obesity is exceeding the expected levels in body weight considering height which is a result of the excessive increase in the body fat relative to lean body mass. The calculation of body density via underwater weighing with the direct body fat measurement method is accepted as "Gold standard." Its implementation is very difficult except the experimental studies. The indirect methods of measuring body fat are listed below:

- Weight assessment according to age;
- Weight ratings according to height;
- Waist circumference measurement;
- Arm circumference measurement;
- Skinfold thickness;
- Body Mass Index (BMI): BMI is an index assessing the body weight based on size and provides information on body fat distribution. It is obtained by dividing Body weight (kg) to squared height (in meters) (kg/m^2).

Body Mass Index (kg/m^2) is calculated as the following: Weight (kg)/Height x Height (sqm) accordingly. In Table 1 WHO classification is shown [66].

It is the most widely used indirect measurement method and accepted worldwide. When height, weight and BMI reference values vary by age and gender, growth curves that are established according to age and gender are used in assessment. Using data from the research in 2007 (Multicentre Growth Reference Study (MGRS)), WHO published WHO MGRSs' growth curves. Children who were breastfed up to 2 years were included in the study. "The" is recommending the usage of "The European Childhood Obesity Group," "International Pediatric Association," "UN Standing Committee on Nutrition" ve "International Union of Nutrition Sciences" WHO MGRS (2007) growth curves. Currently it is used over 100 countries widely. Percentile values are recommended for the evaluation of children and adolescents as an individual and Z-score is highly recommended for the evaluation (SSE) of society [68].

Table 1. Classification of obesity in adults according to the BMI

*Body Mass Index (kg/m²)	Rating
<18.5	Chronic protein energy malnutrition
18.5-19.9	Acceptable
20.0-24.9	Normal
25.0-29.9	Slightly fat
30.0-34.9	1 obese
35.0-39.9	2 obese
>40.0	3 obese (morbid)

*BKI or VKI.

BMI values according to the intersection of z-scores in z-score table are classified as:

- <-2SS "too thin";
- ≥-2SS - <-1SS "thin";
- ≥-1SS - <1SS "normal";
- 1SS- <2SS "overweight";
- ≥2SS "obese" (WHO-MGRS (2007) [68]).

Obesity classification according to WHO BMI:

- Overweight: 85-95 persentile or ≥1 - <2 Standard Value (SS)
- Obesity: ≥95. persentile or ≥2 SS

The Prevention of Obesity

Especially in the last 20 years the significant increase in obesity prevalence causes more individuals struggle with body weight. The fact that there is no effective treatment prevents reaching the target body weight [69]. Generally, gaining kilos is easy and losing weight is difficult. Therefore, it is better to prevent obesity before its treatment. The most important feature in obesity prevention is the application of a diet appropriate to energy balance from an early age [70]. At a young age, especially overfeeding during infancy accelerates the formation of new fat cells. More fat cells are stored by age and this situation makes it difficult to lose weight [71]. For that reason the nutrition of infants and children in a way that they can maintain their energy balance is of great importance in preventing them from obesity. In order to success the individual is required to be trained at an early age about acquiring the right eating habits. However, helping children and young people to gain appropriate physical activity and ensuring them to make a habit of this behavior are also important [72].

It is important to make students calculate their daily energy expenditure and energy consumption in schools in order to give them practical knowledge and help them turn it into habit for leading a life appropriate to energy balance [69]. In a study measuring the impact of nutrition education; it is found that the group that is educated tended to develop positively in menu planning and in the consumption of healthy foods [73]. In the study conducted with 399 students in Los Angeles; it is found that nutrition education changed students' nutrition knowledge, attitudes and habits in a positive way [74].

Conclusion and Recommendations

As a result, obesity at any age has biochemical and physiological effects that could lead to serious health problems. Protection from obesity should start in the perinatal period and continue during the entire life. The development of obesity in older age is assumed to be lower in breast-fed babies compared to babies fed with formula food [75]. When we consider that physical activity and eating habits are taught in childhood, the protection programs should be targeted primarily children and adolescents [76]. Children consume the food that their families buy. Therefore, first step in helping children to have a positive nutritional habit is to prefer foods which are fresh and with low fat and sugar to ready foods. The amount of calories received daily from fat should not exceed 30% of total daily calories.

Meals should be eaten with the family at the table not while watching TV. Foods with calorie such as sweets and chocolate should not be used as a reward [77]. Besides, the implementation of continuous and regular healthy feeding programs in kindergartens, primary and secondary schools or even including them in school curricula is very important in terms of the continuity of struggling with obesity. The positive results of the implementation of nutrition programs in schools have been reported [78]. As well as following a healthy diet within the family, children's sedentary activities such as TV and computer should be limited and they should be directed to physical activities instead. Obesity is not only an aesthetic problem but it is also a problem that can kill. When a conscious society is not formed against obesity, it will be the issue of children at a very young age and obesity rates will go on increasing. In international dimension taking the necessary precautions to prevent from obesity and obesity-induced diseases is recommended urgently. To beat obesity, which has become a public health, the cooperation of family, school and community is very important.

References

[1] Baysal A. Genel Beslenme Bilgisi. Ankara, Turkey: Hatipoglu Publishing House; 1989. p. 7.

[2] Baysal A. Beslenme. Ankara, Turkey: Hatipoglu Publishing House; 1999. p. 13.

[3] World Health Organisation Technical Consultation. Obesity: Preventing and Managing the Global epidemic. Geneva: WHO Technical Report Series; 2000.

[4] obeziteninkardiyovaskulerhastaliklara-etkisi-ve-cocuklukta obezite. Available from: http://www.tkarediyet.com/tr/34/articleCat/2/articleID/33/p/diyetdanismanligi (accessed 01.12.2014).

[5] Bozbora A. Surgical treatment of obesity. *J ANKEM*. 2002; 16(3): 337.

[6] Endokrinoloji ve Metabolizma Hastaliklari Bilim Dali Hasta Bilgilendirme Formu. Available from: http://hastane.omu.edu.tr/saglikli-bilgiler/endokrinbelgeler/%C5%9E%C4%B0%C5%9EMANLIK.pdf (accessed 14.12.2014).

[7] Parlak A, Cetinkaya S. Cocuklarda Obezitenin Olusumunu Etkileyen Faktorler, Antalya; 2006. p.27.

[8] Hedley AA, Ogden CL, Johnson CL, Carroll MD, Curtin LR, Flegal KM. Prevalence of overweight and obesity among US children, adolescents, and adults, 1999–2002. *JAMA*. 2004; 291:2847–2850.

[9] Ogden CL, Carroll MD, Kit BK, Flegal KM. Prevalence of childhood and adult obesity in the United States, 2011-2012. *JAMA*. 2014; 311(8):806-14. doi: 10.1001/jama.2014.732.

[10] Currie C, Nic Gabhainn S, Godeau E, Roberts C, Smith R, Currie D, et al. Inequalities in young people's health. Health Behaviour in School-aged Children international report from the 2005/2006 survey, Health Policy for Children and Adolescents, No.5. Copenhagen: WHO Regional Office for Europe; 2008. Available from http://www.euro.who.int/InformationSources/Publications/Catalogue/20080616_1 (accessed on 17 June 2015).

[11] Whitaker RC, Wright JA, Pepe MS, Seidel KD, Dietz WH. Predicting obesity in young adulthood from childhood and parental obesity. *N Eng J Med*. 1997; 337:869-873.

[12] Serter R. Obezite Atlası, Ankara; 2003.

[13] de Onis M, Blösner M. Prevalence and trends of overweight among preshool children in developing countries. *Am J Clin Nutr*. 2000; 72:1032-9.

[14] Lobstein T, Frelut ML. Prevalence of overweight among children in Europe. *Obes. Rev*. 2003; 4:195-200.

[15] Akıs N, Pala K, Irgil E, Aydin N, Aksu H.. Overweight And Obesity Among 6- 14 Year- Aged Schoolchildren At Six Elementary Schools in Orhangazi-Bursa. *J. Uludag Univ Med Faculty*. 2003; 29(3):17-20.

[16] Suzek H, Ari Z, Uyanik BS. School children in the 6-15 age overweight and obesity prevalence was living in Mugla. *Turkish J Biochem*. 2005; 30(4):290-295.

[17] Karamahmutoğlu, Dirençli Hipertansiyonun Vucut Kitle Indeksi ile Iliskisi, YUT, Istanbul; 2007. s. 26.

[18] Deckelbaum RJ, Williams CL. Childhood obesity: the health issue. *Obes Res*. 2001; 9(Suppl 4):239-43.

[19] Bultman S, Michaud E, Woychik R. Molecular characterization of the mouse agouti locus. *Cell* 1992; 71:1195-204.

[20] Naggert J, Fricker L, Varlamov O. Hyperproinsulinemia in obese/fat mice associated with carboxypeptidase E mutation with reduced enzyme activity. *Nat Genet*. 1995; 10:135-42.

[21] Zhang Y, Proenca R, Maffei M. Positional cloning of the mouse obese gene and its human homologue. *Nature* 1994; 372:425-32.

[22] Maffeis C. Aetiology of overweight and obesity in children and adolescents. *Eur. J. Pediatr.* 2000; 159:35-44.

[23] Gurel FS, Inan G. Childhood Obesity- Diagnostic Methods, Prevalence and Etiology. *ADÜ J. Med.* 2001; 2:39-46.

[24] Kelleher CC, Viljoen K, Khalil H, Somerville R, O'Brien J, Shrivastava A, et al. Lifeways Cross-Generation Cohort Study Steering Group. Longitudinal follow-up of the relationship between dietary intake and growth and development in the Lifeways cross-generation cohort study 2001-2013. *Proc Nutr Soc.* 2014; 73(1):118-31.

[25] Patro B, Liber A, Zalewski B, Poston L, Szajewska H, Koletzko B. Maternal and paternal body mass index and offspring obesity: a systematic review. *Ann Nutr Metab.* 2013; 63(1-2):32-41.

[26] Arslanoglu I. Approach to obesity in children and adolescents. Turkish Pediatrics Archive/Turk Pediatri Arsivi. dec2009, 44(4):115-119. 5 p. 4 Charts. *Pediatri Arflivi* 2009; 44:115-9.

[27] Wabitsch M. Overweight and obesity in European children and adolescents: causes and consequences, treatment and prevention: An introduction. *Eur J Pediatr.* 2000; 159:5-7.

[28] Kelleher CC, Viljoen K, Khalil H, Somerville R, O'Brien J, Shrivastava A, et al. Lifeways Cross-Generation Cohort Study Steering Group. Longitudinal follow-up of the relationship between dietary intake and growth and development in the Lifeways cross-generation cohort study 2001-2013. *Proc Nutr Soc.* 2014;73(1):118-31.

[29] Santaliestra-Pasías AM, Rey-López JP, Moreno Aznar LA. Obesity and sedentarism in children and adolescents: what should be done? *Nutr Hosp.* 2013; 28(Suppl 5):99-104.

[30] Subrahmanyam K, Kraut RE, Greenfield PM, Gross EF. The impact of home computer use on children's activities and development, *Children Comp. Technol.* 2000; 10(2):123-144.

[31] Vandewater EA, Bickham DS, Lee JH. Time well spent? Relating television use to children's free-time activities. *Pediatr.* 2006; 117(2):e181-e191. Available from: www.pediatrics.org/cgi/content/full/117/2/e181.

[32] Nielsen AC. 2001–2002 US Television Household Estimates Report. New York, NY: ACNielsen; 2002.

[33] Patel SR, Hu FB. Short sleep duration and weight gain: a systematic review. *Obes. (Silver Spring).* 2008;16(3):643-53.

[34] Haller R, Rummel C, Henneberg S, Pollmer U, Köster EP. The İnfluence of Early Experience with Vanillin on Food Preference Later in Life. *Chem Senses.*1999; 24(4):465-7.

[35] Schaeffer JP. The lateral wall of the cavum nasi in man, with especial reference to the various developmental stages. *J. Morphol.* 1910; 21:613–707.

[36] Pritchard JA. Deglutition by normal and anencephalic fetuses. *Obstet Gynecol.* 1965; 25:289.

[37] Mennella JA, Ventura AK. Understanding the basic biology underlying the flavor world of children. *Curr. Zool.* 2010; 56(6): 834−841,

[38] Cinaz P, Bideci A. Obezite. Pediatric Endocrinology. In: Hulya Gunoz, Gonul Ocal, Nursen Yordam, Selim Kurtoglu, editors. First Printing, Printing Kalkan. Ankara: Oksoloj Association of Pediatric Endocrinology and Publications 1.; 2003. p. 487–505.

[39] Koksal G, Gokmen Ozel H. Cocukluk ve ergenlik doneminde obezite. Ankara: T. C. Saglik Bakanligi Yayinlari; 2008.

[40] Resch M, Haasz P, Sido Z. Obesity as psychosomatic disease. *Eur Psych*. 1998; 13:315.

[41] Deveci A, Demet M, Ozmen B, Ozmen E, Hekimsoy Z. Psychopathology, alexithymia, and self-esteem in obese patients. *Anatol J Psych*. 2005; 6:84-91.

[42] Karakaya K, Baran E, Tuzun H, ve ark. Turkiye Beden Agirligi Algisi Arastirmasi. Ankara: Saglik Bakanligi, Sagligin Gelistirilmesi Genel Mudurlugu; 2012.

[43] Sujoldzić A, De Lucia A. A cross-cultural study of adolescents BMI, body image and psychological well-being. *Coll Antropol*. 2007; 31(1):123–30.

[44] Kensinger GJ, Murtaugh MA, Reichmann SK, Tangney CC. Psychological symptoms are greater among weight cycling women with severe binge eating behavior. *J Am Diet Assoc*. 1998; 98(8):863-8.

[45] Babaoglu K, Hatun G. Childhood obesity. *Sted*. 2002; 11: 8-10.

[46] Altinkaynak S, Yigit H, Ertekin V. Childhood obesity. *Syndr Med J*. 2002; 14(1): 66-73.

[47] Kannel WB. The disease of living. *Nutr. today*. 1971; 6(3):2.

[48] Goran MI, Davis J, Kelly L, Shaibi G, Spruijt-Metz D, Soni SM, et al. Low prevalance of pediatric type 2 diabetes: where's the epidemic? *J Pediatr*. 2008;152:753-5.

[49] Reinehr T. Clinical presentation of type 2 diabetes mellitus in children and adolescents. *Int. J. Obes. (Lond)*. 2005; 29(suppl 2):S105-S110.

[50] Fagot-Campagna A, Pettitt DJ, Engelgau MM, Burrows NR, Geiss LS, Valdez R, et al. Type 2 diabetes among North American children and adolescents: an epidemiologic review and a public health perspective. *J Pediatr*. 2000;136:664-72.

[51] Liese AD, D'Agostino RB Jr, Hamman RF, Kilgo PD, Lawrence JM, Liu LL, et al. The burden of diabetes mellitus among US youth: prevalance estimates from the SEARCH for Diabetes in Youth Study. *Pediatrics* 2006;118:1510-1518.

[52] Comlekci A. Evaluatıon of cardıovascular rısk ın metabolıc syndrome, and coronary artery dısease. *Turkiye Klinikleri J. Int. Med. Sci*. 2006; 2(3):55-59.

[53] Oguz A. Metabolik sendrom tanimi nedir? In: Oguz A, editor. Soru ve Cevaplarla Metabolik Sendrom. Istanbul: Medya Tower Publishing; 2008. p. 8-13.

[54] Sarti C, Gallagher J. Metabolik sendrom Prevalansi, KKH riski ve tedavisi. *J. Diabet. Comp*. 2006; 2:106-120.

[55] Kang HS ve ark. Low-density lipoprotein particle size, central obesity, cardiovascular fitness, and insulin resistance syndrome markers in obese youths. *Int J Obes Relat. Metab. Disord*. 2002; 26:1030-1035.

[56] Oguz A. Metabolik sendrom. *Psychopharmacol Bull*. 2008; 18(2):57-59.

[57] King DS, Wofford MR. Obesity and hypertension. *Drug Top*. 2000; 3:59-67.

[58] Narkiewicz K. Obesity-related hypertension: relevance of vascular responses to mental stress. *J. Hypertens*. 2002; 20(7):1277-1278.

[59] Swales JD. Manual of Hypertension. Oxford: Blackwell Science; 1995. p. 1-3, p. 119-123, p. 153-160.

[60] Sharma AM, Engeli S. Managing big issues on lean evidence: treating obesity hypertension. *Nephrol Dial Transplant*. 2002; 17: 353-355.

[61] Otake S, Takeda H, Suzuki Y, Fukui T, Watanabe S, Ishihama K, et al. Association of visceral fat accumulation and plasma adiponectin with colorectal adenoma: Evidence for Participation of Insulin Resistance. *Clin Cancer Res*. 2005; 11(10):3642-6.

[62] WHO. Obesity: Preventing and managing the global epidemic. Report of a WHO consultation on obesity. Geneva, June 1997. Geneva: World Health Organisation; 1998. HO/NUT/NCD/98:1.

[63] Bugianesi E: Steatosis, the metabolic syndrome and cancer. Aliment *Pharmacol Ther.* 2005; 22:40-3.

[64] Obezite-ve-solunum-sistemi-hastaliklari. Available from: http://zehirlenme.blogspot.com.tr/2009/07/html(13.12.2014).

[65] Odabasi E. Uyku Apnesi ve Obezite Nedir?. Available from: http://formeo.com.tr/kilo-yonetimi-yazi/158/uyku-apnesi-ve-obezite.html (08.08.2014).

[66] Ng KC, Lai SW. Application of anthropometric indices in childhood obesity. *South Med. J* 2004; 97:566-70.

[67] Çayır A, Atak N, Köse SK. Assessment of Obesity Frequency and Related Factors on Individuals Attending to the Department of Nutrition and Dietetics. *J. Ankara Univ. Faculty Med.* 2011; 64(1):13-19. DOI: 10.1501/Tıpfak_000000779.

[68] WHO. Obesity and Overweight. Geneva: World Health Organisation; 2013. Available from: http://www.who.int/growthref/who2007_VKİ_for _age/en/;http://www.who.int/growthref/VKİfa_girls_5_19years_per.pdf; http://www.who.int/growthref/VKİfa_boys_5_19years_per.pdf (Erişim Tarihi 03.10.2013).

[69] Linde, J. A., Jeffery RW, Levy RL, Sherwood NE, Utter J, Pronk NP, et al. Binge eating disorder, weight control self-efficacy, and depression in overweight men and women. *Intern J Obes.* 2004; 28:418-425.

[70] Baysal, A. Beslenme. Ankara, Turkey: Hatipoglu Publishing House; 2004. p. 495.

[71] Işıksoluğu M. Beslenme MEB. Yayınları. Ankara; 2000. p. 324-325.

[72] Baltaci G, Ersoy G, Karaagaoglu N, Derman O, Kanbur N. Ergenlerde sağlıklı beslenme, hareketli yaşam. Ankara: T. C. Saglik Bakanligi Yayinlari; 2008.

[73] Glanz K, Hersey J, Cates S, Muth M, Creel D, Nıcholls J. ve diğ. Effect of a Nutrient Rich Foods Consumer Education Program: Results from the Nutrition Advice Study. *J Acad Nutr Dıet.* 2012; (112)1:56-63.

[74] Prelip M, Kinsler J, Le Thai C, Erausquin JT, ve Slusser W. Evaluation of a school-based multicomponent nutrition education program to ımprove young children's fruit and vegetable consumption. *J Nutr Edu Behav.* 2012; 44(4):310-318.

[75] von Kries R, Koletzko B, Sauerwald T ve ark. Breast feeding and obesity: cross sectional study. *BMJ.* 1999; 319:147-50.

[76] Cole TJ, Bellizzi MC, Flegal KM, Dietz WH. Establishing a standard definition for child overweight and obesity worldwide: international survey. *BMJ.* 2000; 320:1240-3.

[77] Patient Information Collection: Nutrition. *Am Fam Phys.* 2004; 69:923-39.

[78] Fowler-Brown A, Kahwatı L. Prevention and treatment of overweight in children and adolescents. *Am Fam Phys. 2004*; 69:2591-9.

EDITOR'S CONTACT INFORMATION

Dr. Wenbiao Wu, PhD

Professor

College of Food Science, Southwest University,

Beibei, Chongqing, PRC

Email: wbwu2009@sina.com

After spending 18 years as a research scientist and more than 5 years as a Vice-Director at Southern Potato Research Center of China, Dr. Wenbiao Wu took a position as Professor at Southwest University in 2001 to teach and preside over research in the area of science and technology of foods and food resources with emphasis on food security and toxicology, human nutrition related to interactions of food components with human health and nanotechnology for protein separation. He has published 40 papers, 4 Books and 4 patents, and developed 4 food products that are currently manufactured and sold in market in China. His educational qualifications: PhD in Food Science (University of Reading, UK); BSc in Soil and Agricultural Chemistry (Hua Zhong Agricultural University, PRC).

Index

A

B

C

D

E

F

G

H

I

J

K

L

M

N

O

P

R

S

T

U

V

W

Z